T0201784

Patient and Provider Interaction

Patient and Provider Interaction

A Global Health Communication Perspective

LISA SPARKS AND MELINDA VILLAGRAN

polity

The right of Lisa Sparks and Melinda Villagran to be identified as Author of this Work has been asserted in accordance with the UK Copyright, Designs and Patents Act 1988.

First published in 2010 by Polity Press

Polity Press
65 Bridge Street
Cambridge CB2 1UR, UK

Polity Press
350 Main Street
Malden, MA 02148, USA

ISBN-13: 978-0-7456-4536-0
ISBN-13: 978-0-7456-4537-7(pb)

A catalogue record for this book is available from the British Library.

Typeset in 9.5 on 12 pt Utopia
by Servis Filmsetting Ltd, Stockport, Cheshire
Printed and bound in Great Britain by
MPG Books Group, UK

The publisher has used its best endeavours to ensure that the URLs for external websites referred to in this book are correct and active at the time of going to press. However, the publisher has no responsibility for the websites and can make no guarantee that a site will remain live or that the content is or will remain appropriate.

Every effort has been made to trace all copyright holders, but if any have been inadvertently overlooked the publisher will be pleased to include any necessary credits in any subsequent reprint or edition.

For further information on Polity, visit our website:
www.politybooks.com

Contents

Tables

Acknowledgments and Dedication

We would like to acknowledge and dedicate this book to the following people.

To Daniele (*mi amore*).

My children, Elena, Arianna, and Athena (*mi bugaboos*).

My father, John O. Sparks, who taught me to value education, and who at the young age of 57 fought and ultimately died of lung (primary) and brain (secondary) cancer in 1997.

My mother Marcia Sparks, who is the best listener I know, who supports everything I believe in and try to achieve.

My extended family and all of the precious friends and colleagues along my journey – especially the thoughtful and detailed edits from dear colleague and friend Jim Query and other anonymous reviewers, as well as the savvy insights, flexibility, and unwavering encouragement of Polity publisher and friend Andrea Drugan.

Chapman University President Jim Doti who made this book possible through his unwavering support and commitment to my contributions, as well as Chancellor Daniele Struppa, Schmid College of Science Dean Menas Kafatos, Senior Associate Dean Janeen Hill, Vice-Chancellor Raymond Sfeir, and Associate Vice-Chancellor Jeanne Gunner.

My supportive colleagues at the University of California, Irvine, including Frank Meyskens, Hoda Anton-Culver, Allan Hubbell, Lari Wenzel, Dele Ogunseitan, and numerous others with whom I have had the great pleasure of working over these last few years.

My graduate students in the Master of Science Health Communication program at Chapman University – and above all my research assistant Kat Rogers who provided constructive insights and reliable assistance with this book.

And especially to all the patients and providers, caregivers, and supportive relationships that touch our lives.

Festina Lente!

Lisa Sparks, PhD

To my Mom, Linda Ling, the best doctor, nurse, counselor, patient, caregiver, cancer survivor, and role model I could ever imagine.

Melinda Villagran

Patient and Provider Interaction: Prologue

If you think about it, the very first interaction that most of us ever have is with a health-care provider. Our very first medical encounter happens when we leave the womb, and from our first cry until our last breath we are in the presence of health-care professionals. From birth until death our lives are shaped by the quality of our own health care. *Patient and Provider Interaction: A Global Health Communication Perspective* provides an insightful examination of the important relationship between patients and their health-care providers. The book is written with the understanding that students are also patients, caregivers, and in some cases even health-care providers. As such, this book is written for anyone who has experienced a memorable health-care interaction. The book offers a systematic look at how communication may be used to empower participants in health-care interactions, influence family members, support caregivers, and create meaningful relationships to improve health care in general. A strong communication infrastructure helps patients and providers make the most informed health decisions in an effort to achieve better health outcomes.

Patient and Provider Interaction proposes a systematic approach to help students decide which health-care questions to ask and when, where to get reliable information, and how or when to share the information with others in an effort to save lives. In this book, we explore why effective and appropriate health communication can be a key to achieving optimum health, and/or building a constructive patient and provider relationship. The field of communication is most relevant when it is examined in a context familiar to students, and the patient and provider relationship is just such a context. From a global perspective, this book sheds light on how communication impacts, and is impacted by, the cognitive, relational, cultural, and organizational structures learned in other courses. The global perspective implies that although each dyadic interaction is unique, they all possess certain patterns, opportunities, and challenges for patients and providers. This book helps reveal the patterns of interaction that can positively or negatively impact health outcomes.

Health communication and behavior change

Almost everyone has a memorable story about a health-care interaction. Working in the field of health communication, it is common to hear examples from students about how communication with a provider led to a health-care success, or a health-care nightmare. Often these examples highlight how a communication problem led to a bad decision, a family feud, or a health emergency. At other times the examples center around conflicting or confusing health messages. Newspapers, family members, friends, and health-care providers can have differing ideas about what is healthy, what is risky, and what to do to maintain a healthy lifestyle. Although providers are the most common sources of trusted health information, sometimes even they can have differing opinions about what behaviors are healthy or unhealthy. One provider will say that a certain food is not healthy and should be avoided altogether. Another provider will say the very same food is actually healthy, and should be eaten regularly to avoid (insert your own health-care disaster here). Health communication comes in so many forms and from so many sources, that even the most knowledgeable patients can feel confused about how to make healthy decisions. It is easy to see why patient–provider interactions can be very messy and complex! Examining these issues in the context of the college classroom helps students to understand differing perspectives and develop the skills necessary to weigh various alternatives to make the best health-care decisions.

Health providers play one of the most important roles in influencing patient decision-making in health environments. According to research by the American Cancer Society (ACS), a doctor's recommendation is the best predictor of preventative cancer screening, to give just one example. Patients who participate in regular check-ups with their doctors will be more likely to discover cancer early and, as such, will be presented with more treatment options (Smith et al., 2009). Despite this, patients sometimes avoid honest communication with providers about topics such as current prescriptions, health history, or potentially risky lifestyle choices. There is no denying that ineffective, incomplete, or unsatisfactory patient and provider interactions have a negative influence on health outcomes.

This book seeks to provide specific information about how to avoid common problems in the provider–patient relationship. As a student, this topic will help you more deeply explore many familiar communication topics and experiences from your own life, and do so in a way that helps you more fully understand the links between the scholarship and the practice of communication in real-world contexts.

What is *your* approach to your health interactions? Do you have a tendency to ask a lot of questions? Do you find yourself gathering as much information as possible when you experience something new, or do you ask questions in a situation in which you don't fully understand what is happening? Do you sometimes find it difficult to communicate with and to completely understand people who are from a different background than you? We hope so – because if you answered "yes" to some or all of these questions, *Patient and Provider Interaction: A Global Health Communication Perspective* is the right book for you. We also realize some people understandably choose to actively avoid communication about health because they fear it will lead to uncertainty or sadness. The fact is everyone is born, and everyone dies, and in between we all face health challenges. In difficult life moments it is our hope that this book may offer you hope or solutions to dealing with challenging health issues. Communication is a powerful tool to help heal bumps and bruises received in the past. The misunderstandings and miscommunication that occur in health interactions can be just as damaging and traumatic as biological illness, and patient–provider interactions can affect your life in dramatic ways.

We wrote this book in honor of those who value the power of effective health communication and choose to study it in the college classroom. We wrote it in part because we have been studying and researching this topic for more than 25 years combined, but also because we have "been there" as caregivers and patients ourselves. We understand that the patient and provider relationship is both unique and familiar; both complex and understandable. Students will recognize a variety of interpersonal communication topics in this book because the patient and provider relationship provides a context within which a wide range of interpersonal communication issues occur. Students may have studied intercultural communication, but not how culture permeates the way patients experience health care. And students may have studied organizational communication, but never considered how health organizations are similar or different from other organizational types. The patient and provider relationship is a microcosm of many communication contexts and as such supplies a useful lens through which to look at communication in a new way.

While we have made our own unique contributions to the literature provided and have drawn upon our expertise in our writing of *Patient and Provider Interaction*, we have also drawn upon the expertise of numerous scholars with whom we have collaborated, and from whom we learned about this topic, based on their research. We want to take this opportunity to recognize all of the health communication and public health scientists who have made this work richer and more useful for our readers. The goal of *Patient and Provider Interaction* is to lead the reader through the maze of tasks and information that influence patients and families as they deal with health issues for the first time. We also want to offer a deeper knowledge of the importance of communication processes, and highlight how such knowledge can lead to better health outcomes. Finally, it is our greatest hope that this book will also offer insights for health-care providers searching for some additional evidence-based insights about how to maximize patient satisfaction, positive health outcomes, and most effectively and appropriately communicate with and build relationships with their patients.

About the chapters in this book

Patient and provider interaction (PPI) is a major focus of health communication. The first chapter provides a basic introduction to PPI through an overview of health communication as a central component of behavior change. PPI is defined from a perspective grounded in health communication theory and research, and involves creating shared meaning about health care and conditions in the medical encounter. PPI is viewed as an extremely effective context for health behavior change. Strategic interaction in PPI can be effective in disseminating important and credible health information.

Chapter 2 offers discussions of the increasingly important topic of health literacy and discusses how becoming health literate can lead to better health outcomes through improved cultural competence, oral and written communication, and numeracy. Patients and caregivers alike must become literate consumers of health information by increasing their knowledge and ability to communicate about important health topics. The goal is to be able to work with your health-care provider team by playing a powerful role in the decision-making process.

Chapter 3 pays particular attention to patient characteristics and information management by exploring the ways in which such goals are based on information needs such as seeking and avoiding, social support, uncertainty management, knowledge, attitudes, beliefs, behaviors, and agency, as well as the lay theories patients often have about their health and the health-care system.

Chapter 4 focuses on health-care providers and their characteristics. Providers are often a great source of reliable information about every stage of health care. Health-care providers tend to answer most questions about the illness itself, but often are not equipped to deal with patients' varied informational, emotional, and psychological needs. Because the relationship between health-care providers and patients is quite complex, we pay particular attention to the role of friends and family, as well as nurses, social workers, physicians' assistants, laboratory technicians, and all aspects of the health-care team (in addition to the physician).

Chapter 5 outlines the importance of caregiving by examining the communication needs of patients and caregivers, issues of hospice and palliative care, social support, and communication issues related to end-of-life decision-making, death, and dying. In addition, this chapter pays particular attention to emerging aspects of the distance caregiving context.

Chapter 6 considers the impact of cultural influences on patient and provider interaction. Culture creates a context for communication and a set of rules or norms for the ways in which we talk about health-care and conditions. We describe how culture shapes patient and provider values and beliefs about health, expectations for visits, knowledge, attitudes, organization of the health-care system, and societal and cultural norms about what it means to deal with illness and make health decisions. Culture permeates every part of our world and therefore also has a tremendous impact on health-care processes.

Chapter 7 explores how health issues shape and often change an individual's social identity. This chapter provides an intriguing discussion on how a health diagnosis (e.g., cancer) changes the ways in which people talk and relate with other people. For instance, how do patients, family members, and friends deal with identity shifts from living a life not involving cancer, to cancer often becoming a dominant part of the overall identity?

Chapter 8 focuses on the role and influences of social media technologies, and how these can impact patient and provider interaction. Health-care consumers of all ages use various technologies to obtain health information and communicate with providers. Similarly, friends and family share health concerns and talk with each other about health issues every day. Interactive technology, e-health, and online communication have opened the way for individuals to create and maintain social networks by linking patients, providers, and family members to health organizations, as well as increasing knowledge about health care. And providers are utilizing technologies in unprecedented ways, from text messaging to databases to surgery.

Chapter 9 examines effective patient and provider communication within health-care organizations, emphasizing the role of health-care teams' approaches in helping to coordinate the mixed messages that patients and their families often face as they navigate the complex health-care environment. Health organizations that are more effective at balancing the tasks and relationships in the group usually have members who are more satisfied, more team-oriented, and as a result more effective at maximizing the potential of health-care delivery leading to better health outcomes.

Chapter 10 provides a conclusion to the additional communication issues that are likely to arise in the patient and provider interaction, including various aspects that may not have been covered or that may need more attention. This chapter is an epilogue of sorts that provides a conversational approach to the ideas behind the book.

The good news is that health care is much improved from how it was just a few decades ago, which has resulted in greater numbers of individuals living through their seventies and beyond than ever before in history! This means we are all likely to have an increased number of health-care interactions as we age and live longer, healthier lives. As a result of picking up *Patient and Provider Interaction*, you are more informed and possess the skills to take action in the daily life choices in front of you, and, as such, can make better health choices and decisions along your health-care journey. The health-care experience is often a balance between hope, confusion, and sometimes despair, and our goal is to help readers feel a little more hopeful about their powerful role in the health-care communication process as it impacts their health decisions and experiences. *Patient and Provider Interaction* provides a comprehensive, rigorous, but accessible approach to understanding the important relationship between providers and patients, and shows how such crucial information exchanges, and subsequent informed decision-making, not only can produce more satisfactory health interactions but also can increase health outcomes.

Knowledge and competence are incredibly powerful. So, too, is communication, which can play a huge role in prevention. The role of communication is equally significant in terms of its effect on the health decisions we make before, during, and after a serious health diagnosis.

After reading *Patient and Provider Interaction*, we truly believe that you will have another important tool to draw upon, whether you experience the health-care setting every day as a provider, or encounter its complexity for the first time as a patient, student, or caregiver. Although there may be challenges along the health-care journey, and during some health-care interactions, you will have useful tools to deal with the obstacles with more confidence, as well as information to guide you through the complications and difficulties you will indeed encounter. We make health choices through communication. We create, maintain, and destroy relationships through communication. We hope that by reading *Patient and Provider Interaction,* you will be better equipped to deal with the various health messages and relationships in your life, thereby producing better health outcomes for yourself, your family, and friends. We hope that in some small way, by using the communication tools acquired by reading *Patient and Provider Interaction* your own experiences with the health-care system will avoid the difficulties described in the following pages. *Festina Lente!*

PART I

INTRODUCTION TO PATIENT AND PROVIDER INTERACTION

1 Patient and Provider Interaction: Introduction

Send and Receive
"It's only a little spot."
I have cancer.
"We can get it all out."
They're going to crack my chest.
"The radiation only produces a little sunburn."
My neighbor got fried.
"The chemotherapy isn't bad."
My mom barfed for days.
"It's just a small shadow on your spine."
I'm going to be paralyzed,
I'm going to have pain.
"It seems to have spread to your liver
But there is this new drug –"
I'm going to be a guinea pig,
I'm going to die.
One fact,
one reality.
Two truths.
One sent,
one received.

Frank L. Meyskens, Jr, MD, FACP

"Send and Receive" was written by a physician who experiences provider and patient interaction in the difficult and emotional health environment of cancer care. The basic sender–receiver model taught in many communication courses is applied to a realistic situation where messages about illness are sent and received in very different ways. The facts are the same, but the perspective and meaning of the interaction are very different for the patient and the provider. Social conventions prevail when the sender and receiver choose their words wisely, in part to represent an intended meaning, and in part based on each person's experiences and perspective.

When this poem was read at a gathering of health-care providers and researchers, for many providers in the room it summarized the complexity of their professional experiences talking with patients. For others, the poem resonated as a reminder of emotional conversations with their own provider, or the health-care providers of a loved one. Difficult conversations about difficult health topics are among the most memorable conversations in our lives, and the study of patient and provider interaction offers a chance to explore how to improve the quality of the messages that are sent and received. Students who explore the challenges of patient and provider interactions may then develop the skills necessary to approach the situation in the best possible manner. Communication is complex, and the study of patient and provider interaction also allows teachers and students to share their own experiences as they delve more deeply into the components of successful communication with a provider.

Like teachers and students, most communication between patients and providers seeks to achieve shared meaning. Effective and appropriate health communication, also known as competent communication, is a central aspect of quality health care across the continuum of care from detection, diagnosis, treatment, survivorship, and end-of-life. Health care provides an excellent context for the study of communication because it transcends the college classroom by aiding students with the knowledge and skills necessary to build supportive health-care relationships throughout the life span. Relationship-building is the core process of competent communication, and by studying patient and provider interaction, students will learn the essential skills necessary to build supportive health-care relationships. It is not enough for patients and providers – informal as well as formal – to enter into this important set of relationships without a desire to connect with each other, which builds trust and mutual admiration and will ultimately lead to a better understanding of each other as well as an increase in effective health decisions and subsequent outcomes.

Patients must be able to tell their story to their providers and providers must have a goal of obtaining the most complete story possible, and to achieve this must understand the language and the emotions, the verbal and the non-verbal aspects of each interaction.

This book uses the term "provider" to refer to anyone in the field of health care who renders aid to patients and caregivers. Providers include such professions as doctors, nurses, speech therapists, physical therapists, laboratory and X-ray technicians, hospital personnel, home health-care workers, midwives, complementary and alternative medicine providers, and emergency medical technicians. Each of these relationships is grounded in the need for trust, openness, and competent communication. In patient and provider interactions with all types of health-care professionals, conversation and non-verbal cues are used to create shared meaning.

During conversation, patients and providers deliver communicative cues – via **narratives**, **self-disclosure**, and often through **humor** – that give the savvy listener hints about their goals (Sparks, Travis, and Thompson, 2005). Each person in the interaction must engage in **active listening strategies**, and follow up the detection of such communicative cues with **conversational selection strategies** such as "yes, go on," "I am listening," "uh-huh," and probes such as "so you were saying X, can you explain what you mean by that specifically?" or "I am intrigued by X, can you tell me more about that?" Both parties must begin moving away from an anxiety-producing model of health communication and move toward a model of putting each other at ease with the freedom to talk to each other about often delicate and personal issues that arise in health-care interaction. A central feature of all communication is that questions impact answers. The way a question is framed or structured influences the resulting response. Although medical training and decision trees often call for close-ended questioning when it comes to talking with patients, as in all relationship-building communication more **open-ended question formats** will elicit longer and more thorough answers. Longer answers may be less efficient in the short run in terms of time, but more efficient in the long run, because they provide more evidence and information to make a successful diagnosis and treatment plan. Evidence about the nature of the patient's illness can then shape future interactions, and more effectively focus the conversation to improve health outcomes.

Evidence-based research and practice is important and essential, but is not enough. In addition to the use of the intellect and informed health communication skills, patients and providers must tap into their intuition and insights, pay careful attention to details that emerge in interaction, and engage in active listening in each health-care encounter. It is also important to understand that individual interactions are influenced by a history of interaction. In other words, a patient may have already seen a number of providers who have not been able to explain what is wrong and why. Such patients may come to the interaction with a high level of frustration due to their past experiences within the flawed health-care system. Effective and appropriate health communication practice must complement evidence-based practice. This book is an attempt to unpack the varied and complex aspects of patient and provider interaction from a crucial and somewhat distinctive health communication theory and research-based approach.

Defining patient and provider interaction

Patient and provider interaction, as defined from a global perspective grounded in health communication theory and research, involves **creating shared meaning** about health care and conditions in the patient and provider encounter. Shared meaning is essential to competent communication, but it is not always easy to achieve due to differences in language, culture, and experiences. Patients come into each medical encounter for a variety of reasons, and typically have specific goals for their medical visits. Unfortunately, sometimes patients leave the interaction without achieving their communication goals. For example, in the US, as many as 25 percent of patients leave medical visits feeling their questions have not been answered, but only about 11 percent of patients in the UK feel their goals have not been met (Davis et al., 2006). Despite these differences, all patients seek to understand their health better after a visit to a provider and to use communication with their provider to create shared meaning and increase understanding.

The patient and caregivers' goals may be obvious based on visible symptoms, or more obscure if the problem is not easily diagnosed in a single examination. Sometimes a patient may even have a different goal from their caregiver parent or adult child. Patients and their caregivers have time schedules, financial pressures, and unspoken perceptions, and each of these factors can play a role in the provider and patient interaction. Providers, too, come to the medical encounter with specific goals. The provider also has time schedules, financial pressures, and unspoken perceptions, but each of these factors may be quite different from those of the patient. Together, the provider, patient, and caregiver interact, based on their individual goals, in an effort to create shared meaning that (hopefully) succeeds in achieving the best possible outcome for all parties. This book includes separate chapters on the characteristics of patient, provider, and caregiver that shape the patient and provider relationship.

The powerful role of **culture** and **identity** in the patient and physician relationship also has an important impact on different experiences in medical care. Diverse voices come from diverse backgrounds, and each person's social and cultural identity is formed based on the racial, ethnic, gender, socioeconomic, educational, and geographical groups to which they belong. Culture and identity play important roles for both patients and providers. Think, for example, how a foreign-born female provider might view her work in a health-care clinic in the Midwestern US quite differently from such work in a clinic in her home country. Think how her patients might view this provider differently from the way they would a male physician who was born in the local community. Who we are impacts on the way we interact, and culture and identity are at the core of many decisions about communication. We will cover both of these topics in further detail in our chapters emphasizing such varied background and often socially constructed characteristics.

Patient and provider interactions increasingly include mediated forms of communication such as email or text messages, and they almost always occur within the structure of a larger health organization. Rules and norms that govern what, how, and whether to communicate with patients inside and outside the clinic are rapidly changing, based on advances in technology and changes in the health delivery system (Wagner, 2010). Some physicians take it upon themselves to create innovative approaches to communication with patients such as YouTube and Twitter, while others rely on channels provided by their health-care plan such as magazines or quarterly reports. We cover the theory and practice of health organizations and communication technology in the separate chapters of this book.

How can health communication theory inform what we know and do not know about patient and provider interaction in the medical setting? First, we must have a basic understanding of what the field of health communication can offer us, based on how it has evolved since its inception in the late 1980s. We can then learn about the way health communication theory and research influences every aspect of the patient and provider encounter. Patient and provider interaction (PPI) is a major focus of health communication. PPI is viewed as an extremely effective context for health behavior change. Strategic interaction in PPI can be effective in disseminating important and credible health information.

Health communication to enhance behavior change

Health communication provides the foundation of provider and patient interaction. As such, it is important to lead with a precise definition of health communication: "health communication involves creating shared meaning about health care and conditions" (Sparks, 2010: 2). The US Department of Health and Human Services (2000), in achieving the Healthy People 2010 initiative to educate the public on the nation's major health priorities, put forth this definition of health communication:

> The art and technique of informing, influencing, and motivating the individual, institutional, and public audiences about important health issues. The scope of health communication includes disease prevention, health promotion, health care policy, and the business of health care as well as enhancement of the quality of life and health of individuals within the community.

Health communication covers a wide-ranging array of topics, including disease control and prevention, emergency preparedness and response, injury and violence prevention, environmental health, workplace safety, and general communication behavior as it relates to well-being and leading healthy lives. Health promotion efforts at the national level often take a developmental life-span perspective with a focus on adolescent health, aging, women's health issues, men's health issues, school health, and minority health (Parrott, 2004).

An important JCAHO report in 2002 revealed, "root cause analysis finds more than 80 percent of medical errors are due to communication breakdowns" (p. 2). It is clear that patient and provider interaction encompasses an important set of communication variables that we must better understand from an evidence-based perspective grounded in theory and research.

As we will describe in further detail in our chapter on provider perspectives to PPI, provider communicator style can greatly impact the patient and provider relationship. Research indicates that communication interventions to improve quality of care should target both providers and patient communicative behaviors (see, e.g., Epstein et al., 2007; Sparks 2007/2008). In addition, research reveals physicians are more patient-centered with patients they perceive as better communicators, more satisfied and compliant (Street, Gordon, and Haidet, 2007).

Research indicates that active patients tend to be more satisfied and compliant patients with higher levels of health literacy (Street et al., 2005). Research also shows that patient-initiated active participation behaviors occur 84 percent of the time, with active patients revealing higher levels of education and Caucasian female patients revealing more negative feelings and concerns than their male counterparts (Street and Gordon, 2005).

Female physicians were found to use more supportive talk than their male counterparts, and physicians were found to use less supportive talk with non-Caucasian patients (Street et al., 2005).

Further, patient and provider interaction includes a wide range of providers beyond the physician. Patient and provider interaction also includes family members, friends, companions, caregivers, and health-care providers, ranging from nurses to other medical personnel connected with the patient's care. Companions also play a crucial role in patient and provider interactions, although participation levels of the companion vary greatly (see, e.g., Street and Gordon, 2008; Street et al., 2008). The patient and provider relationship is enhanced when patients see themselves as similar to their providers, in terms of communication as well as beliefs and values (Harwood and Sparks, 2003; Sparks and Harwood, 2008; Villagran and Sparks, 2009). Findings indicate perceived personal similarity to be linked with higher ratings of satisfaction, trust, and medical adherence (Street et al., 2005).

It is clear that health-care providers have followed a number of traditional approaches to health care that often leave patients and family members unsatisfied with their care. The **biomedical model of medicine**, which is an evidence-based approach to medicine that relies on scientific methods and procedures for verifying disease, tends to favor a focus on the patient as a cell rather than a human being. This approach can accurately diagnose causes of symptoms and subsequent treatment regimens, but it is not the best approach in terms of patient-centered care. **Patient-centered care**, rather than focusing primarily on physical causes of illness, takes into account the important **physical and psychosocial** aspects of illness including cultural beliefs, attitudes, norms, and coping abilities, as well as life events that may interact with and/or complement physical health problems. Patient-centered care has been defined as "providing care that is respectful of and responsive to individual patient preferences, needs, and values and ensuring that patient values guide all clinical decisions." (IOM, 2001) adopted the saying "Nothing about me without me" to signify the importance of patients' voices in their own medical care.

By conveying a sense of the broadened scope of health communication theory and research, this book is intended to unpack provider and patient interaction based on the communication that creates the interaction. As such, this book takes a different perspective from other books on patient and provider interaction, that are typically written by physicians or others in the medical community, because we consider the science and the art of medicine as co-equal pieces of health care. In other words, biomedical science about symptoms of illness are important features of every medical encounter, but awareness and shared meaning about those symptoms only comes into existence through the process of communication. Our overarching purpose is to provide and shed light on such complex health-care encounters by offering an evidence-based health communication framework through which health-care interventions might occur in patient and provider relationships. To achieve this goal, we begin this chapter with a brief discussion on the state of science in health communication theory and research, and how it is impacting and influencing provider and patient interaction. This section includes an overview of the major variables in health communication research that influence patient and provider interaction.

The state of health communication research

The field of health communication has grown exponentially over the last 25 years or so (Beck, 2001; Thompson et al., 2003), with research in health communication becoming one of the most highly regarded contexts of communication study among communication professionals. There are currently two journals devoted to the topic of health communication: *Health Communication,* published since 1989 by Lawrence Erlbaum Associates, and *Journal of Health Communication,* published since 1996 by Taylor and Francis. Scholars have also discussed the history, future trends, and specific contexts in health communication in several overview books (see, e.g., Beck, 2001; du Pré, 2001, 2005a; Geist-Martin, Ray, and Sharf, 2003; Jackson and Duffy, 1998; Kreps and Thornton, 1992; O'Hair, Sparks, and Kreps, 2007; Sparks, O'Hair, and Kreps, 2008a; Thompson et al., 2003) and special issues of journals (see, e.g., Parrott, 2004; Ratzan, 1994; Sparks, 2003b), as well as hundreds of journal articles and book chapters. All have provided important outlets for the study and dissemination of health communication research, policy, and practice. Through these works, health communication scholars are dramatically increasing attention to pertinent health communication issues and contributing in important ways by translating such research into policy and practice. Because of the inherent complexities of contemporary health communication and the potential to impact on society, we must continue to clearly disseminate the most important theoretical and methodological orientations of the health communication field. There is no better way to inform the health-care and research community than to engage in translating such research efforts into practice.

At its core, the health communication field focuses on two major elements: (1) message production and processing; and (2) the creation of shared meaning about health issues in relationships. Communication researchers and professionals address myriad health-care issues from a variety of perspectives, including interpersonal and relational issues in provider–patient communication, breaking bad news, communication and skills training, disclosure issues, caring for special populations such as older adults, broader social and community health issues, such as prevention, health-risk communication and strategic communication approaches to care, cultural issues and disenfranchisement, social support, social identity issues, health organizations and decision-making, health information sources, health campaigns, the role of spirituality, the role of humor, narratives, interviewing and message strategies in health care, health literacy, information technologies, e-health, and telemedicine, as well as broader health policy issues (for a detailed account of the history of health communication, see Thompson et al., 2003).

In addition to research on messages and relationships, health communication scholars focus on evaluating the effectiveness of patient–provider interaction and health campaigns. Research has generated increasing understanding of how to stimulate desired health behaviors via communication (see Sparks, 2007/2008; Sparks and Turner, 2008; Wright, Sparks, and O'Hair, 2008; Witte, 1998). However, such theory-driven and evidence-based health communication interventions must be continually evaluated for effectiveness and adjusted accordingly. If such evaluations reveal that certain variables are not receiving the consideration needed, then new, theoretically based interventions can be developed to improve health outcomes.

In an era in which access to health information has a profound effect on longevity, one important health communication research goal, especially of the National Network of Libraries of Medicine (NN/LM), has centered on improving health-care provider access to health information, especially in rural, under-served, and minority communities (see Witte, 1998). In recent years, the health literacy movement, with links to health communication, policy, and practice, has extended this commitment to health information access for all, as evidenced by the National Academy of Sciences, National Library of Medicine (NLM), Healthy People 2010 and the Institute of Medicine (IOM) (see Kreps and Sparks, 2008; Sparks and Nussbaum, 2008). As Thompson (1984) acknowledged, it is important to investigate variables that moderate processes, discovered in prior research, and then build upon those studies in new investigations rather than starting from scratch.

Implications for patient and provider practice, education, and research

The purpose of this chapter was to provide an introduction to patient and provider interaction. Effective and competent communication in the patient and provider interaction is a key component in bringing about behavioral change, which is what truly matters.

To influence entrenched health behaviors, messages need to be relevant and compelling, with health information providing direction and rationale to enable the best health-related decisions and adoption of health-preserving behaviors (Maibach, Kreps, and Bonaguro, 1996; Kreps and Sparks, 2008). Care must be taken to coordinate content and relational aspects of communication in order to inform people about cancer and cancer treatment without confusing or upsetting them (Buckman, 1996; Gillotti, Thompson, and McNeilis, 2002; Sparks and Villagran, 2009). This book is an attempt to shed light on the importance of the varied and complex communication issues that exist and influence patient and provider relationships, from a global perspective grounded in health communication.

2 Health Literacy

In a 2009 interview with Oprah Winfrey, Patrick Swayze's widow, Lisa Nieme, commented that her IQ dropped 50 points when she heard the word "cancer" as her husband was diagnosed for his illness. This brought a big flashback for me. I had a similar situation when I ended up in the emergency room after a fall. I was seen by three doctors and it felt like each one was speaking a different foreign language with terms like "lumbar vertebrae" and "transverse fracture." I was thinking to myself, "what happened to my graduate degree and my English fluency?" You're in a white robe, cold and in pain, reverting to thinking in your native language (Spanish in my case) and simply terrified. The last "doctor" who saw me happened to be a resident and I had complimented his jade ring. He told me; "It was a gift from my mom," and I added, "She must be very proud." He left, saw me crying and came back. He: (1) drew a picture of the spinal cord highlighting the lumbar vertebrae; (2) told me that I didn't need a cast and that with time, I would be able to go to work and carry my child; and (3) Yes! – I was getting pain medication shortly. These were the three key messages I needed to hear right away with a culturally sensitive and hopeful tone.

E. Natal, personal communication, November 16, 2009

Health literacy is an emerging and extremely important area of communication around the world. The topic of health literacy as an important health communication issue has been receiving national and international attention during the last few years. Even among patients in European countries with nationalized health-care systems who have more access to care than residents in other parts of the world, there are still people who struggle to read, understand, and use information essential to preventing a trip to the doctor in the first place. Some health-care communication researchers argue that in order to improve the usability of health information, there must be improvement in the usability of health services, coupled with increased knowledge and better relationships in an effort to improve decision-making. These components can then be used to bolster health literacy outcomes within organizations (US Department of Health and Human Services, 2010). This is essential because health literacy has emerged as an important issue in recent years, and it affects the health outcomes of individuals.

Health literacy is an important construct for understanding patients' needs for health information, as well as their abilities to access and utilize such health information and messages for critical health decision-making. Currently, health literacy is defined by the National Academy of Sciences,

National Library of Medicine (NLM), Healthy People 2010, and the Institute of Medicine (IOM) as:

> the degree to which individuals have the capacity to obtain, process and understand basic health information and services needed to make appropriate health decisions that may affect the health of Americans and the ability of the healthcare system to provide effective, high quality care.

As such, patients need to be able to competently locate and then evaluate health information for credibility and quality, to analyze relative risks and benefits, calculate dosages, interpret test results, and so on. Health literacy includes the concepts of accessing and understanding information and services, with a comprehensive skill set of literacy that potentially includes **visual** (graphs and charts), **computer** (operate and search), **information** (obtain and apply relevant information), and **numeracy** (calculate and reason numerically) skills required to make appropriate health decisions (see, e.g., Nielsen-Bohlman, Panzer, and Kindig, 2004; Ratzan et al., 2000). Further, patients need strong **oral communication skills** to adequately and accurately describe their symptoms and concerns, and to enable them to competently search for and understand health information to strengthen decision-making skills. The highly scientific nature of much health information makes an understanding of basic scientific method also important.

According to the American Medical Association, poor health literacy is "a stronger predictor of a person's health than age, income, employment status, education level, and race" (*Report on the Council of Scientific Affairs*, Ad Hoc Committee on Health Literacy for the Council on Scientific Affairs, American Medical Association, JAMA, February 10, 1999). In *Health Literacy: A Prescription to End Confusion*, the Institute of Medicine reports that 90 million people in the United States – nearly half the population – have difficulty understanding and using health information. As a result, patients often take medicines on erratic schedules, miss follow-up appointments, and do not understand instructions such as "take on an empty stomach." Furthermore, the US Department of Education (2007) reports that age is a predictor of lower health literacy, with 59 percent of patients over 65 and 70 percent of patients 75 and older having basic or below-basic health literacy skills. However, health literacy issues are not limited by demographics. In fact, we can all benefit from clear, simple communication and non-intimidating access to health care (J. McKinney, personal communication, November 6, 2009).

Health literacy includes the ability to understand instructions on prescription drug bottles, appointment slips, medical education brochures, doctors' directions and consent forms, and the ability to negotiate complex health-care systems. Health literacy is not simply the ability to read. It requires a complex set of reading, listening, analytical, and decision-making skills, and the ability to apply these skills to health situations. The definition of health literacy can also be expanded to include providers and their "capacity to communicate clearly, educate about health and empower their patients" (R. S. Owens, personal communication, November 6, 2009). Danielle Ofri, a New York City physician, supports this definition in a blog post:

> I see the doctor as a translator. For most people, medicine is a foreign country, with its own language customs, and mores. My patients are immigrants to this country, and many feel very disoriented. My job, as their physician, is to translate this alien world for them, to help them acclimatize and hopefully thrive. (2009)

Health literacy varies by context and setting and is not necessarily related to years of education or general reading ability. A person who functions adequately at home or work may have marginal or inadequate literacy in a health-care environment. With the move towards a more "consumer-centric" health-care system as part of an overall effort to improve the quality of health care and to reduce health-care costs, individuals need to take an even more active role in health-care related decisions. To accomplish this, people need strong health information skills. Health literacy may be described as based on four elements:

1 cultural and conceptual knowledge,
2 listening and speaking (oral literacy),
3 writing and reading (print literacy), and
4 numeracy (knowledge of statistics and other numeric data used in healthcare).
   (DHHS, 2010; IOM, 2004)

Although recent developments, including analytics and health information technologies, are allowing providers to better tailor their services to individual patient needs, many physicians continue to take a more routine approach to medicine and patients (McGee, 2009). Research indicates that physicians who pay attention to aspects of health literacy tend to communicate better with their patients. Similarly, the health literacy of patients has been shown to impact the patients' perceptions of the information given by the provider (Ishikawa et al., 2009).

Literacy impacts health knowledge, health status, and access to health services. Health status is influenced by several related socioeconomic factors. Literacy impacts income level, occupation, education, housing, and access to medical care. The poor and illiterate are more likely to work under hazardous conditions or be exposed to environmental toxins (National Network of Libraries of Medicine, 2010).

The Center for Plain Language focuses on health literacy by posing the following questions. Do we live in a society where people can:

1 find what they need;
2 understand what they find; and
3 use it to accomplish their goals?

If you were to ask yourself these same questions, would you consider yourself to be proficient and comfortable in navigating the health-care environment? This chapter hopes to accomplish the following goals:

1   to help you to understand the emerging and important research area of
    communication science and literacy; and
2   teach you how you can increase your health awareness and
    understanding.

Thus, you will increase your health literacy so you can make more informed
health decisions and achieve better health outcomes.

Health literacy is defined as the degree to which individuals have the
capacity to obtain, process, and understand basic health information and
services needed to make appropriate health decisions. Only 12 percent of
adults have proficient health literacy, according to the National Center for
Education Statistics (2003). In other words, nearly 9 out of 10 adults may
lack the skills needed to manage their health and prevent disease. And
14 percent of adults (30 million people) have below basic health literacy.
These adults are more likely to report their health as poor (42 percent) and
are more likely to lack health insurance (28 percent) than adults with proficient health literacy. Low literacy has been linked to poor health outcomes
such as higher rates of hospitalization and less frequent use of preventive
services.

Health literacy can greatly impact patient safety and health outcomes.
The IOM (2001) defines patient safety as "avoiding injuries to the patients
from the care that is intended to help them," and communication between
providers and patients is essential to avoid these errors. Unfortunately, the
Joint Commission on Accreditation of Healthcare Organizations (2002)
claims that more than 80 percent of medical errors are caused by communication breakdowns that may be due to literacy issues. Health literacy
typically deals with an individual's ability to navigate the health system, to
obtain clinical information, and to obtain information about preventive
activities, although in recent years the definition has been broadened to
include institutions, systems, and communities, in addition to individuals.
Health literacy should not be defined purely on the individual level in terms
of a person's knowledge, but should also include the greater community's
ability to provide spaces for people to participate in healthy lifestyles and
to provide opportunities for creating shared meaning and understanding
through communication among all community members.

In other words, it is not just an individual's responsibility to cook
healthy meals and go to the gym or boot camp. It is also the community's
responsibility to create attractive open spaces with trouble-free access
and admission to biking, hiking, and running trails, as well as to increase
access to healthy stores. Further, the community can and should provide
places where people can more easily get check-ups for their own health
needs. For instance, for cancer protection and prevention behaviors,
community leaders can teach new parents about the importance of
putting sunscreen on their young toddlers every day and, as a result, these
parents can then show their growing children how to put sunscreen on
every day. Such a simple prevention behavior could become an embedded health behavior for these fortunate children. Community leaders can

offer healthy shopping and cooking events and/or a model for implementing a healthy living plan within each neighborhood or community association.

Health literacy is increasingly recognized as an important issue affecting communication across the continuum of health care. Recent research shows that, upon receiving diagnoses of diseases such as cancer and Alzheimer's disease, patients and their families often face decisions for which they are unprepared (Alzheimer's Disease Education and Referral Center, 2007). Surprisingly, health-care providers and the medical establishment are often equally unprepared to help patients and their families make the best and most informed decisions. Health communication scholars increasingly report that treatment choices are often made in an environment of uncertainty, ambiguity, misinformation, high emotion, and anguish, so the outcome ends up being less favorable than recent medical advances could enable (ADERC).

Patients can improve health literacy

The saying "nothing about me without me" refers to the need for patients to gather, process, and articulate their feelings about credible health information in making decisions with providers about health care (Berwick, 2002). This is difficult for individuals with low socioeconomic status, as access to health information is more limited within this group (Houston and Allison, 2002). Regardless of income or education, health literacy can be quite confusing and daunting. Patients must come to health-care situations prepared with as much credible information as possible. They should also enter the health-care setting with questions prepared to ask their doctors. It is helpful to write them down beforehand. The health-care system can be a maze of misinformation. Moreover, health information can vary by source. When the US Preventative Services Task Force announced in 2009 new recommendations for mammograms, suggesting that women wait until age 50 to begin breast cancer screenings as compared to the previous recommendations to begin at age 40, the National Cancer Institute responded by including the new guidelines in recommendations to doctors and the public (Sack and Kolata, 2009). However, many doctors decided to continue to suggest screening at age 40 for their patients, saying that early detection is more important than reducing the number of unnecessary tests for many women (Belluck, 2009). Another controversial subject among health providers and pharmacists is the use of generic medications. While many pharmacists and providers suggest that generics are identical to name-brand medications, studies have shown that generics can differ by up to 20 percent from the name-brand, having the potential to cause side-effects in sensitive patients (L. Rohret, personal communication, December 15, 2009). Patients should therefore seek out information from a variety of sources to make well-informed decisions that suit their individual health needs.

Printed consumer health-care materials delivered to patients in multiple countries may have inaccurate or improper word translations. While discussing the difficulties of creating accurate health information, drug company executives complain that there is no "generic" Spanish that everybody can understand. When you write something in Royal Academy Spanish, you end up with something totally incomprehensible to most people in Mexico or Latin America. Peter Intermaggio, a senior marketing communicator for Comcast, has similar frustrations: "An essential truth of the Hispanic market is that information is obscured by language difficulties and poor translation" (as cited in Wentz, 2009). In Spain, a computer is an *ordenador*. To the rest of the Spanish-speaking world, a computer is a *computadora* and an *ordenador* is a very mean person who gives orders to you. So, if you tell a Latin American that they must use their *ordenador* to find information, they will think that they must get help from their very mean assistant principal. A non-profit organization is an organization *sin animo de lucro* in Spain. *Animo* means spirit in Spanish, and in some cultures you must be careful to avoid invoking spirits. Moreover, most don't know what *sin animo de lucro* means. Offering health information can be very difficult unless one knows how to translate health information. One needs to become familiar with the linguistic and cultural choices of the community. Most drug companies and worldwide health-care companies make efforts to ensure that information is accurate, but, as a consumer, it is important to be careful when translating information from Internet chatrooms or other informal channels.

In other words, it is the job of health consumers to arm themselves with as much information as possible, and to be savvy consumers of that information. Not every source is a good source. There is a need to consider who wrote the information. Gathering information is the first step, but analyzing the information to consider inconsistencies is the next step. It is vital not to take every piece of information at face value. That is certainly not to say one should doubt all information, but, rather, remain aware that there are choices to be made about which information is viewed as credible for each situation.

When reading health information or talking to health authorities, it is important to understand that statistics about a particular health issue may apply to a demographic group, and not be related to a specific individual. Each patient has different characteristics that may result in a stronger health outcome (e.g., overall physical health status, genetic predispositions, tolerance for certain medications and treatments). However, it is not surprising that people who simply look at the numbers associated with a certain disease often lose hope, give up, and even die without any real knowledge in terms of how they would have responded to certain treatment options that could have resulted in them gaining several years of life or more. Because health literacy is such a complex issue for patients, a variety of patient and caregiver advocacy groups, such as the American Kidney Foundation and the American Lung Association, have been formed in recent years in an effort to raise awareness about particular diseases.

Imagine the following scenario:

> A friend has just been diagnosed with cancer, and the friend needs help gathering various kinds of health information about cancer by talking with doctors and other health-care providers, as well as through online searches. Even with a college education and significant online research skills, it is tough to wade through all the general information available online and in the media that does not seem to relate to the friend's situation. Even by processing a mountain of information, and sorting through the different and sometimes conflicting findings from different cancer studies and various websites, specific and credible information is not available. Searching for hours and even days to find exactly the right information is a process that takes considerable research skills. Even when credible information is available, often the information is difficult to understand because it uses technical language, with new definitions and ways of talking about the diagnosis, possible treatment options, as well as conflicting research on the topic.

Physicians helping patients improve literacy

As health educators, physicians help their patients build health literacy. The relationship between the patient and physician can influence health, functioning, and satisfaction (Zoppi and Epstein, 2002). In one study, Stewart et al. (2000) reported that once patients perceived they had reached common ground with their physicians, outcomes improved; patients experienced more satisfaction, decreased concern, and fewer requests for referrals to other physicians. Many researchers have provided tips that physicians can follow in order to improve communication. Zoppi and Epstein recommend active listening, helping patients tell their stories, and increasing patient participation in the decision-making process. Other important steps that physicians can follow are to understand a patient's experience, build partnership, provide evidence, present recommendations, and finally check for understanding (Epstein, Alper, and Quill, 2004). If a patient is not complying with the physician's requests, the provider should ask the patient about barriers to adherence and concerns specific to the treatment in order to address concerns that are unique to the individual (N. Ali, personal communication, November 15, 2009). Ensuring that the patient participates, is informed, and understands the process and options can be very helpful because it increases both satisfaction and health.

Information is important

Current health literacy processes go beyond the initial definitions or topics related to obtaining, processing, and understanding basic health information and services. Gathering and processing such important health information is a crucial first step, but acting on this information in order to make informed choices and improve one's health and behaviors across the life span is usually the ultimate goal. Health communications must seek to not only provide the materials but also deliver them effectively and ensure that they are helping patients implement change in their lives. Creating easy-to-understand messages is merely the first step in a much more complicated process toward behavioral change (J. McKinney, personal communication, November 13, 2009). It is not as easy as setting up a strong argument and targeting a population to change health behavior. People may have the knowledge, but still choose the unhealthy path (e.g., lack of sunscreen protection; etc.). Why is this? We need to better understand the impact of cognitions *and* emotion, considering how they can strongly take hold of behavioral decisions no matter how irrational such decisions may be (e.g., smoking, excessive drinking, not using a condom).

Mental processing and feelings

From very early in life, humans are constantly bombarded by messages that demonstrate what is later perceived to be normal or normative behavior. Normative behavior is what is considered by most of those individuals around us to be acceptable behavior (i.e., within the norm). For instance, children who grew up in an environment where there was a heavy amount of drinking, smoking, drugs, deception, heavy TV viewing, lack of vegetables in the daily diet, and no sunscreen protection will likely grow up to view those behaviors as normal or normative. A "script" for how to behave is created based on a person's sex, cultural orientation, nationality, religion, and age. We all draw upon those scripts to make decisions about whether a certain behavior is risky, or healthy. For example, in the US, cousin marriage is often viewed as non-normative or unhealthy, but in many European countries royal families have been marrying their cousins for centuries. On a day-to-day basis, decisions about wearing condoms, breastfeeding babies, skydiving, taking medication, visiting herbal healers, and a variety of other risky or healthy behaviors are driven by whether they are perceived as normative among each person's reference group.

Young teens may choose to not use a condom during sexual intercourse because they see TV shows of young people having unprotected sex, and rarely does a television show demonstrate the potential aftermath of unprotected sex (STD, HIV) as part of the plotline. The fact is that main characters in television shows do not often get STDs, but rarely we will see a more expendable character (in the two-episode special) contract an STD before they are rewritten off the show. Despite this, statistics show that contracting a sexually transmitted disease is quite common and young people are not often literate about the true health implications of unprotected sex. In 2006, the United States received reports of 358,366 cases of gonorrhea and 1,030,911 incidents of Chlamydia. In fact, more than one in five Americans – 45 million people – are infected with genital herpes. Sexually transmitted diseases (STDs) remain a major public health challenge in the United States. While substantial progress has been made in preventing, diagnosing, and treating certain STDs in recent years, CDC estimates that approximately 19 million new infections occur each year, almost half of them among young people aged 15 to 24 (Centers for Disease Control and Prevention, 2009). STDs are a risky business, but they are still viewed as infrequent and non-normative even though the statistics clearly demonstrate how prevalent STDs really are in some age groups. Health literacy can make a difference in the cognitive and emotional impact of these important health decisions and the choices people make in their everyday lives.

How the health-care environment impacts literacy

With a clearer understanding of cognitions and emotion in terms of how they often impact behavioral choices, it is also important to consider how to attain credible information to enable well-informed health-care choices. Health-care providers are the best source of health information, and being honest about risky behaviors may open the door to dialogue that can increase literacy for patients. Health-care providers and health-care systems must create an improved environment in which they can work with patients to create shared meaning that is tailored to each patient.

Health literacy is more than being able to obtain and process information and services. Health literacy is not something patients have or do not have, but instead something that they must improve. Health literacy is, for example, when a health-care provider ensures that a patient leaves their office able to explain their diagnosis, treatment protocol, and/or set of issues in their own words. Health literacy is when providers offer multiple messages in multiple mediums for the message receiver (aka: patients, family members, friends). For instance, when a health-care provider must break bad news to the patient, s/he can talk about it verbally, while also providing a large font written/visual/aural/picture version of the discussion for the patient and his or her caregivers to take home. Additionally, an interpersonally based patient navigator system (much like the teacher–student relationship) could be provided outside of a provider appointment where patients can talk in more detail to clarify their needs and get further information in a variety of appropriate formats. They can therefore have choices in terms of preferred information gathering, understanding, and processing.

Health organizations are now working to raise awareness among providers about the challenges for patients with low literacy. The goal of these efforts is to give providers first-hand experience with health literacy and engage them emotionally in its difficulties. Both short videos that depict the struggles of patients with health literacy and interactive exercises that simulate low-level reading skills have been effective in increasing empathy in providers (J. B. Bryant, personal communication, December 7, 2009). Provider awareness of health literacy is especially important since research suggests that providers commonly overestimate their patients' literacy levels, especially with minority patients (Kelly and Haidet, 2007). Further, many providers do not recognize low literacy as a predictor of patients failing to adhere to recommended treatments, resulting in frustration (Powell and Kripalani, 2005). If patients do not understand their providers' recommendations, they will not be able to follow them properly.

A new program in the United States is aimed at helping hospitals nationwide to determine their patients' communication needs and to implement specific tools to meet those needs. For instance, a hospital in New Jersey has set up a visual picture system of health care that is working. They have created multiple panels of images that provide patients with an opportunity to point to icons showing their specific health issue (e.g., pain or breathing problem) as well as the part of the body that feels different. Patients can also point to their native language in a list so an appropriate interpreter can be identified and brought in to aid in the interpretation of complex health information. Moreover, in Spain, for instance, education and social class are often considered to be major influences on health literacy (Sparks and Villagran, 2008/2009). As such, improvements in health literacy must include these factors to plan effective health communication programs, create improved health outcomes, decrease costs, and increase patient satisfaction. Patients with little education might benefit from the use of a picture system or other tools to help simplify the identification of complex health concerns.

Even with an awareness of health literacy, providers often complain that they do not have the time or the ability to address these needs when dealing with their patients. A recent national study found that although pediatricians are aware of health-literacy related problems and the need for communication with families, they often struggle with time demands in utilizing their skills (Turner et al., 2009).

What does health literacy mean for patients?

Patients are overwhelmed with the vast amounts of information they are exposed to throughout the often lengthy process of discovering they have a serious illness, along with understanding the specific diagnosis, treatment options, and the related outcomes. Literacy means having a basic understanding of a range of health topics and being able to differentiate different types and what these mean in terms of decision-making for better health outcomes. And literacy must include an understanding of basic numbers and percentages, also known as numeracy skills. This can include understanding how to measure doses, how to decipher nutrition labels, how to calculate premiums, co-pays, deductibles, or how to choose a health plan. What can a patient or caregiver do to improve their health literacy? First of all, they can ask their provider simple but specific questions such as: "Can you show me any pictures?" Research supports the notion of patient understanding of health information via pictures in terms of increasing both understanding and recall of health information (see, e.g., Sparks and Nussbaum, 2008; Wright, Sparks, and O'Hair, 2008). Once the health-care provider shows pictures, it is possible to probe further with additional questions to obtain more specific, important information (Sparks, Travis, and Thompson, 2005). For instance: "In this brochure you've given me, could you show me the most important thing for me to do next?" This can be followed by a request for the provider to mark the important areas on the brochure. Another way that health literacy can be increased in the provider–patient interactive environment is by a spouse or a family member accompanying the patient. Ideally, this patient navigator should be a family member or friend or someone a person trusts, who can assist in navigating the health-care maze. Such a person might give reminders of the patient's questions or concerns, and will also listen to the provider's answers. This person can help in identifying specific additional questions that may need to be asked of the provider, so it is clear exactly what has to be done next. Patients often have numerous procedures to undergo, as well as multiple medications that must be administered and taken. For these situations, the savvy patient can ask a simple but specific question such as: "Could you show me how to do that?"

Disparities in health literacy

Vulnerable populations often have significant health literacy difficulties and are challenged by intercultural communication barriers to accessing and making sense of relevant health information. Patients from such populations are often confused and misinformed about health-care services, early detection guidelines, disease prevention practices, treatment strategies, and the correct use of prescription drugs, which can lead to serious errors and health problems. These populations with the lowest levels of health literacy are likely to be poorer and less educated than populations with higher health literacy. Research indicates that better-educated adults are much more likely to search for information on the Internet, whereas less- literate adults are not (Baker et al., 1996; Kripalani et al., 2006; Paasche-Orlow, Schillinger, Greene, and Wagner, 2006; Kutner, Greenberg, Jin, and Paulsen, 2006; Wolf, Parker, and Ratzan, 2008). Less-literate adults have reduced access to computers and the Internet, and decreased capability in terms of reading and comprehending information (e.g., Wolf, Parker, and Ratzan, 2008; Wright, Sparks, and O'Hair, 2008). Thus, while the Internet can be a valuable source of health information, one also has to be mindful about those who have difficulties accessing the Internet.

Environment and community support

Now, imagine that an individual's health literacy knowledge is at a high level, and that the person knows it is important to eat fruit, vegetables, leafy greens and fiber; exercise every day; and get dental check-ups, and other check-ups for cancer prevention (i.e., colonoscopy, mammogram). Having the knowledge may be a first step toward leading a healthier life, but that does not mean a person will have the skill or ability to take action in terms of healthier eating, daily exercise, regular dental check-ups, and regular colonoscopy and mammogram appointments, etc. For example, if someone lives next to an oil rig or near a polluted river in a neighborhood with easy access to fast-food and convenience stores, that person will be less likely to go jogging every day or to eat much farmers' market produce, low-fat dairy products, extra virgin olive oil, and so on. Thus, increasing an individual's knowledge certainly does not guarantee healthier behaviors and lifestyles.

Another barrier to health literacy concerns the delivery of most health information under stressful conditions and circumstances during a particular diagnosis and prognosis; the resultant intense emotion and arousal impacts an individual's ability to process the message being delivered. The step from cognitive processing and understanding to implementing concrete action that embeds healthy behaviors in daily life is a missing link that each individual and family must fill in their own unique way, but community leaders can assist in the process by paving the way toward educating their community one neighborhood at a time. Government and community leaders can help, not hinder, by creating and promoting health literacy interventions that can be easily implemented in communities, while also using tools to measure the health literacy of a community.

Research has shown the significance of health literacy, as well as the importance of patient–provider communication and its positive impact on health outcomes. Findings from the US Department of Education (2007) survey reveal that large numbers of adults are constrained in their ability to use everyday print materials with accuracy and consistency.

How can a patient feel about his or her level of health literacy? The list below shows a few aspects of health literacy that are worth considering when navigating the complex and often confusing health-care environment.

1 How would you define health literacy and describe its importance for health-care environments?
2 How well can you discuss the significance of patient–provider communication and its specific importance related to issues of prevention, detection, diagnoses, and treatment; survivorship, and/or end-of-life?
3 Do you have the ability to evaluate specific efforts to improve patient–provider communication?
4 Do you have the ability to implement concrete techniques that can be employed by patients to improve communication with health-care providers?
5 Can you adequately describe the provider's role in supporting patient (or caregiver) communication with health-care providers?
6 Can you identify specific actions and opportunities that are available to cancer care providers to support patient and caregiver communication with health-care providers?
7 To what extent can you support clients to be better patient communicators with their health-care providers?

Useful websites to aid in health literacy

<http://www.todocancer.com/esp>
<http://www.nia.nih.gov/HealthInformation/Publications/TalkingWithYourDoctor/>

<http://www.nlm.nih.gov/medlineplus/talkingwithyourdoctor.html>
<http://imsersomayores.csic.es/index.html>
<http://www.askme3.org/>
<http://www.aeccjunior.org/>
<www.4women.gov/Tools>
<www.centerforplainlanguage.org>
<http://www.ahrq.gov/questionsaretheanswer/index.html>
<http://www.ahcpr.gov/consumer/quicktips/doctalk.htm>
<http://www.nationaljewish.org/disease-info/symptoms/questions.aspx>
<http://familydoctor.org/online/famdocen/home/pat-advocacy/healthcare/837.html>
<http://www.air.org/naal>

Predictors of poor health literacy

According to the American Medical Association, poor health literacy is "a stronger predictor of a person's health than age, income, employment status, education level, and race" (*Report on the Council of Scientific Affairs*, Ad Hoc Committee on Health Literacy for the Council on Scientific Affairs, American Medical Association, JAMA, February 10, 1999). In *Health Literacy: A Prescription to End Confusion*, the Institute of Medicine reports that 90 million people in the United States, nearly half the population, have difficulty understanding and using health information. As a result, patients often take medicines on erratic schedules, miss follow-up appointments, and do not understand what seem to be straightforward instructions such as "do not take with alcohol, may cause nausea," or "take once a day" which may be confused by Spanish speakers, resulting in an overdose, because "once" may be interpreted as the number 11 in Spanish.

Vulnerable populations include:

- Elderly (aged 65+): two thirds of US adults aged 60 and over have inadequate or marginal literacy skills, and 81 percent of patients aged 60 and older at a public hospital could not read or understand basic materials such as prescription labels (Williams, MV. JAMA, December 6, 1995).
- Minority populations.
- Immigrant populations.
- Low income: approximately half of Medicare/Medicaid recipients read below the fifth-grade level (<http://www.medicarerights.org/main contentstatsdemographics.html>).
- People with chronic mental and/or physical health conditions.

Reasons for limited literacy skills include:

- Lack of educational opportunity: people with only high-school education or lower.
- Learning disabilities.
- Cognitive declines in older adults.

- Use it or lose it: reading abilities are typically three to five grade levels below the last year of school completed. Therefore, people with only a high-school diploma typically read at a seventh- or eighth-grade reading level.

The relationship between literacy and health is complex. Literacy as a term applies to health-care settings, but typically is used more generally as in assessing abilities to read, write, and carry out basic arithmetic. General literacy is a basic requirement to function adequately in today's society, yet 25 percent of the US population is functionally illiterate. Low literacy is disproportionately evident among minorities, those with lower socioeconomic status, and those who have not completed high school (Kutner et al., 2006). In the US, 15 percent of Whites have less than a high-school education as compared to 20 percent of Asians, 28 percent of African-Americans, 29 percent of Native Americans, and 48 percent of Hispanics or Latinos. Reading skills are important when accessing health care, as many health materials are written at the college level, well above the recommended level of fifth grade. For patients to be able to obtain and understand complex information and messages about cancer and treatment (e.g., risks and benefits, informed consent, odds in prognosis, median survival rates), they need above-average health literacy, general literacy, and math skills (Davis et al., 2002).

Health literacy indicates the extent to which an individual has the ability to verbally communicate familiarity and comprehension of technical health and science information, navigating the health-care system, and relational agency (O'Hair and Sparks, 2008). Health literacy impacts health knowledge, health status, and access to health services. Health literacy appears to be an important factor for health-care knowledge, usage, screening rates and medication adherence (Davis, et al., 2002; Davis, et al., 2006; Kreps et al., 2008a; Kreps and Sparks, 2008; Sparks and Nussbaum, 2008). Individuals with low literacy often have increased difficulty understanding details of treatment and decision-making, and may not be able to easily articulate what is needed in the way of further information (see, e.g., Rudd, 2007). Even when simplified materials are made available, patients still may not be able to comprehend them (Coyne et al., 2003; Davis et al., 2002; Kaphingst et al., 2005).

In the US Department of Education (2007), 41 percent of Hispanic, 25 percent of Native American, and 24 percent of African-Americans had below-basic health literacy, as compared to 9 percent of Whites and 13 percent of Asians (Kutner et al., 2006). An individual with below-basic health literacy does not have the skills to circle the date of a medical appointment on a hospital appointment slip or to perform simple arithmetic. Such limited health literacy has been associated with difficulty understanding informed consent documents (Gotay, 2001), lower screening rates (Davis et al., 2001/2002), poorer medication adherence and prescription label comprehension (Davis et al., 2006; Parker and Davis, 2006), increased rates of hospitalization (Baker et al., 2002), higher mortality (Baker et al., 2007;

Rudd, 2007), and less awareness of general public health (Wolf, Parker, and Ratzan, 2008).

Health status is influenced by several related socioeconomic factors. Literacy impacts income level, occupation, education, housing, and access to medical care. The poor and illiterate are more likely to work under hazardous conditions or be exposed to environmental toxins. Individuals at risk for low levels of health literacy are less-educated, elderly, poor, and typically have chronic diseases (e.g., Kutner et al., 2006; Wolf, Parker, and Ratzan, 2008).

Health treatments are often complex and involve patients and family members in numerous decisions. Patients with limited health literacy may be unable to obtain or understand important information about their treatments, which may negatively impact health outcomes such as treatment adherence and frequency of hospitalizations (Sentell and Halpin, 2006). Moreover, many technical health-care contexts such as cancer require patients to have above-average math skills to understand the risks and benefits of treatment, odds in prognosis and median survival rates, as well as for understanding accurate dosage, medication labels, and frequency of medication administration (Parker and Davis, 2006; Davis et al., 2002; Webb et al., 2008). Patients and their family members need a complex set of health literacy skills to optimize the patient's treatment experiences. These skills include the ability to communicate, listen, remember appointments and instructions, ask for clarification, self-advocate, analyze risk factors and negotiate with insurers or health-care providers (see Kreps and Sparks, 2008; Kutner et al., 2006; Sparks and Nussbaum, 2008).

Identifying patients' health literacy levels creates the opportunity to provide better information at appropriate levels to patients at critical and vulnerable times. This in turn should improve patients' understanding of the disease and treatment, and ultimately health-care outcomes. In addition to health disparities that affect access to therapies and survival, there are disparities in accessibility to and utilization of pertinent health-care information. Often the individuals most in need of interventions are those who are the hardest to reach or have the least resources. Overall, ethnic minorities, low-income populations, and individuals with low health literacy do not have equal access to the relevant information necessary to navigate the health-care system and obtain optimal care (Safeer and Keenan, 2005). Evidence suggests that information is more likely to be retained when messages are tailored and timed to coincide with patients' needs and skills (Bandura, 1997).

The Office of Disease Prevention and Health Promotion (2006) report emphasizes the need to clearly identify causal factors for disparities in care, so that interventions are developed to remediate these factors. There is growing evidence concerning the mediational role that health literacy plays in the access to and utilization of health care as well as the production of health disparities, which have huge public health implications (Wolf, Parker, and Ratzan, 2008).

Wolf, Gazmararian, and Baker (2007) examined the relation between health literacy and health risk behaviors in a sample of adults, aged 65 years and older. Results showed that individuals with marginal or inadequate health literacy scores tended to be older, be Hispanic or African-American, and have lower levels of education and lower income. Low health literacy, however, was not associated among this sample with health risk behaviors, such as heavy drinking, cigarette smoking, and having a sedentary life-style. Another study conducted by Wolf, Gazmararian, and Baker (2007) showed that Medicare enrollees with inadequate levels of health literacy had lower physical function and mental health than those with adequate health literacy levels, after controlling for chronic illness incidence, health risk behaviors, and demographic variables. A study conducted by Baker et al. (2007) investigated health literacy levels in relation to overall and cause-specific mortality in a sample of 3,260 Medicare enrollees. Results showed that inadequate health literacy predicted all-cause mortality in the study. Further, fluency in reading was the most influential factor in explaining the association between SES and health status. Wolf et al. (2005) developed a reliable and valid measure of patient self-efficacy with cancer patients and found that literacy-related items, including understanding and participating in care, maintaining a positive attitude, and seeking and obtaining information, were important mediating factors of cancer care. These findings could inform the patient and provider interaction in important ways.

Information seeking

The National Cancer Institute (NCI) Cancer Information Service (2005) has identified that there are demographic differences in information requests received by their call center (Rutten, Squiers, and Hesse, 2006): Hispanic cancer patients more often requested information about psychosocial support than did Whites; more information seekers had some college education or above; older patients were more likely than younger patients to seek information about disease; and women were more likely than men to seek information (Rutten, Squiers, and Hesse, 2006; Squiers et al., 2005; Ramanadhan and Viswanath, 2006). General patient barriers to obtaining information include psychological adjustment to diagnosis and treatment, (Barsevick, 2002; Sparks, 2003a; Sparks, 2008; Sparks and Turner, 2008), cultural differences (Collins, Villagran, and Sparks, 2008; Pecchioni et al. 2008; Sparks and McPherson, 2007), communication with providers (e.g., Sparks and Villagran, 2008, 2010; Villagran and Sparks, 2010; Wright, Sparks, and O'Hair, 2008), age differences and coping (Folkman et al., 1987a,b; Sparks, 2003a; Sparks, 2008; Sparks and Turner, 2008), coping styles and emotion (Folkman and Lazarus, 1987; Sparks and Turner, 2008), and low literacy (Kreps and Sparks, 2008; Kreps et al., 2008a; Paasche-Orlow, 2005; Sparks and Nussbaum, 2008).

Interestingly, individuals with basic health literacy are more likely to receive their health information from radio and television than are individuals with intermediate or proficient health literacy (Kutner et al., 2006). Individuals with higher levels of health literacy are more likely to use multiple sources, such as the Internet, and personal contacts. They also are more likely to request information from health-care professionals (Kutner et al., 2006).

Discussion Questions to Improve Health Literacy

Patients can improve their health literacy by asking specific questions of their provider. The following Ask Me 3 model suggests that three specific questions can help patients better understand their diagnosis and what they need to do to follow up with treatment. Even if the provider has answered these questions in general, it is always a good idea to ask more questions if information is still unclear in any of these areas.

What is my main problem?
What do I need to do now?
Why is it important for me to do this?

PART II

CHARACTERISTICS INFLUENCING PATIENT
AND PROVIDER INTERACTION

3 Patient Characteristics

Dear Fellow Patients,

Since I'm not quite as formally educated or experienced on this subject as the rest of you, I have a question about what to expect from my doctor. I am constantly frustrated by the types of information I receive and the way it is written, and I was wondering if any of you have ever been in the same position.

When I go to the doctor, I'm often handed printed materials or asked to fill out forms that I'm tempted to rewrite or redesign, then hand them back to doctor or nurse. As a writer, I've seriously considered doing this (even at the risk of making them mad at me) but so far I have been able to resist. My question is, is there a persuasive but polite way to make suggestions to health-care providers about the way they write their materials? Some of the forms I have read before a surgery or during a treatment make me cringe. How can I make recommendations for simple changes? I don't want to come across as a know-it-all because I don't know it all, and also because such an approach or attitude would not help me in the long run. I just want basic information that is understandable and honest.

Here's an example: during my pregnancy, I was referred for a diagnostic ultrasound because of my "advanced maternal age," and because I had decided against a diagnostic amniocentesis. A few days after the procedure I got a form letter about the results. The first four paragraphs talked about Down Syndrome, telling me the definition, risk factors, "markers," and so forth, and how women with "advanced maternal age" are at greater risk to have babies with Down Syndrome. In the fifth paragraph, it explained that my ultrasound was negative for all of the Down Syndrome markers and my baby was fine. Of course by that time I already assumed my unborn baby had Down Syndrome, so I was freaking out completely. It took over a page of writing to tell me my tests were negative. That should have been the lead!!

Just out of curiosity, I ran a software program on the form letter that assesses writing style of documents. The software program told me the document was poorly written, poorly organized, and written above a 12th grade level. When I mentioned this experience to my own doctor, he responded, "Yeah, it's too bad these uneducated people can't read nowadays." I agreed and said, "It's also too bad some educated people can't *write* nowadays." I guess that probably wasn't the best response for building collaboration and support, but since I'm pregnant, I'm blaming hormones. I guess my real question is, "If I want to participate in my own health care is it too much to expect for the provider to use clear written and verbal communication? I guess I am not always clear either, but then again I'm not a 'trained professional.'"

Anonymous, online chatroom for expectant mothers, 2008

One thing that is almost always certain about being a patient is that almost everything is uncertain. We think we know how to spot the signs of illness, comfort a friend after a negative diagnosis, or read a form given to us by our physician, but uncertainty occurs in health care when the information we receive is not clear, not credible, not available, or not accurate (Brashers, 2001). People may want to know the facts about their chances of getting specific diseases, but may feel even less certain about the future if they find out those chances are very high. Sometimes the way information is presented creates uncertainty, and sometimes the information itself is inconclusive or contradictory. For example, expensive genetic testing helps some people gain information about whether they carry a gene that increases the chance of developing different types of cancer. Once the tests are in and the information is available, does having the answer always bring peace of mind to the person being tested? If a test reveals that someone has a 99 percent chance of getting Alzheimer's disease, does the possession of more information encourage more, or less, certainty about the future?

For some people, it is better to know and be able to plan, but for other people more information is not necessarily better. In fact, many people actually fear having too much information about potential illnesses and diseases for which there is no cure. Sometimes it is easy to downplay the importance of information because of the source, or the way it is presented.

In the field of communication, we used to think all communication was about reducing uncertainty (Berger and Calabrese, 1975; Berger and Kellerman, 1983), but in recent decades many communication scholars have moved to the idea that we *manage* uncertainty either by seeking information or by avoiding information regarding our health (Brashers, 2001; Babrow, Kasch, and Ford, 1998).

Communication scholars such as Dale Brashers, Austin Babrow, and Richard Street all focus on the role of information management in patients' decision-making and participation in medical interactions. The fact is that patients are the central focus of health care, and information management plays a fundamental role in the health-care process.

Instead of a natural tendency to reduce tension by increasing knowledge of a given situation, Brashers and colleagues explain that *uncertainty management* means making choices based on the perceived threat of gaining knowledge that is not favorable. When the perceived threat of certain information is high, we may seek out contrary information to *increase our uncertainty* and reduce the threat (Brashers et al., 2000). If, for example, a doctor tells someone she is very confident he or she has less than one year to live, that person might choose to get a second opinion with the hope that the new doctor might say something different and therefore increase the uncertainty about his or her impending death. If the first doctor is certain a person will die, doesn't the existence of differing information help him or her hold on to hope? Unlike the more traditional view of communication as an exercise in uncertainty reduction, uncertainty management dictates that increased uncertainty is often preferable when a threat is high (Brashers et al., 2000). Second opinions can actually reduce anxiety, either by confirming the original diagnosis or by enabling hope for a better outcome (Harpham, 2009). Patients' information needs and the way we manage information about illness impacts our communication with providers, and can ultimately improve our health outcomes.

Much of the work on uncertainty management and information needs of patients builds on the ideas of Mishel (1988). Mishel's *uncertainty in illness theory* describes how uncertainty is created when patients have little or no knowledge or experience with their illness (Mishel, 1988; Mishel and Braden, 1988). Symptoms are unfamiliar to the patient, so the physical manifestations of illness do not trigger a clear understanding of their meaning. For example, if I do not know that dehydration can cause headaches, when I get a headache I don't think, "Maybe I should drink some water." Instead, I feel uncertain about the meaning of my headache and worry it could be something more serious. I cannot make informed decisions or ask the right questions if I do not fully understand the meaning of my situation. I therefore feel uncertain about what to say or do.

When we feel uncertain, we use resources in the environment to gather important health information. Resources used to understand and interpret symptoms of illness include the Internet, discussions with our providers, friends, and family, religious and cultural beliefs, and available print or video materials. Health information is a critical resource that typically comes from successful health communication through a variety of sources (Kreps, 1988, 2003; Pecchioni and Sparks, 2007; Sparks, forthcoming). Effective and timely communication enables patients and their families to gather relevant facts about significant threats to health, and helps them identify strategies for avoiding and responding to these threats (Kreps, 2003; Kreps et al., 2008a).

Health communication researcher Austin Babrow developed *problematic integration theory*, which helps to explain how people engage in information-seeking behaviors and how they manage uncertainty when coping with illness. This theory helps to describe reasons why people may or may not be persuaded by information they receive from a provider, or by information from others that is contrary to what a provider has said. Since uncertainty has a major impact on patients in health-care crises, problematic integration (PI) theory (Babrow, 1992, 1995, 2001) provides an explanation of multiple uncertainties that may coexist on multiple levels (Hines et al., 2001).

Babrow (2001) argued that the meaning of uncertainty is largely dependent on the values of the individual experiencing an illness, and those values guide the ways that information is used to manage uncertainty. For example, a person with MS may decide to gather certain types of information about the most experimental treatment options if he or she places a high value on trying to control the disease, regardless of the side-effects of the treatment. Another person might be more concerned with acquiring information that enhances the immediate quality of life with MS, regardless of the long-term prognosis. In both cases, the values of the patient impact the way information is used to deal with the illness.

PI theory includes two components used in producing and coping with subjective uncertainty: *probabilistic orientations*, the likeliness of the event/issue occurring in their life; and *evaluative orientations*, an assessment of the potential outcome. Babrow (2001) defines probabilistic judgments as "associational webs of understanding that we form through more or less thoughtful engagement with the world" (p. 560). Probabilistic orientations are based in cognition whereas evaluative orientations are based in emotion.

Probabilistic and evaluative judgments can be linked to each other, and can also be reciprocally related. A central claim in PI theory is that an individual's judgments regarding probability and evaluation are often integrated even when they are incompatible with each other. According to Babrow (2001: 554), "expectations and evaluations are interdependent in complex ways." The difference between probabilistic and evaluative judgments is rather like the difference between thinking with the heart or the mind. Relatives may know the outlook for their loved one with a terminal disease is not good, but may still choose to avoid talking about the person's impending death. Cognition and emotion are both powerful influences on the way we communicate, and they can work together or separately to influence our interactions. Sometimes, while we cognitively know it is important to go ahead with a final conversation with a dying loved one, we just might not be emotionally capable of facing the situation. In cases like these, cognition and emotion intertwine to create complex decisions about how and whether to approach the conversation.

For some people, probabilistic judgments may even create the desire to increase uncertainty about an event (Bradac, 2001). For example, we might not think the likelihood of developing skin cancer is high, so we choose not to pay attention to factual information on the topic. Sometimes, even if statistics predict a high likelihood of getting skin cancer, we choose to avoid the topic to manage any potential impact on our day-to-day life. The decision to avoid important information about a health risk can lead to statements such as "I just don't really know if tanning beds cause skin cancer," or "I'm not sure if only tanning a couple times a week is really that dangerous."

Babrow (2001) describes four conditions when it is especially difficult, or problematic, to integrate probabilistic and evaluative judgments:

1 when the two types of judgments diverge from each other;
2 when the probability of occurrence of a threat is ambiguous;
3 when conflicting evaluative judgments (or competing emotions) create ambivalence; and
4 when the outcome of a threat is impossible or unavoidable (and therefore in either case certain).

Examples like this highlight the central role of communication in PI theory in that it can address the uncertainty experienced as a result of health messages. PI theory helps us understand how and why patients, providers,

Table 3.1 Types of problematic integration

Form of problematic integration	Definition	Example
Divergence	A discrepancy between what we want to happen, and what is likely to happen.	I know people with infertility have a hard time conceiving, but in my heart I just know we are meant to be parents.
Ambiguity	The probability of the event/issue is unknown or uncertain.	I have to believe exercising every day will reduce my chances of getting heart disease.
Ambivalence	Mental conflict caused by choosing between two equally valued or mutually exclusive alternatives.	I feel both hopeful that my cancer has not spread, and fearful that it has spread.
Impossibility	The realization that the outcome of an event is certain and inevitable.	Everybody dies some time so why not live now? If I get AIDS from having unprotected sex at least I will know how I will die.

Source: Sparks and Villagran (2010)

and family members generate expectations and make decisions about health care. Ultimately, communication is the source of problematic integration as well as a resource for coping with uncertainty. Communication and decision-making are easier when probabilistic and evaluative judgments merge. In other words, decisions are easier when there is consistency between what people *think* about an illness, and how they *feel* about it. Relying too much on either logic or emotion makes decisions harder because the impact of choices is not fully considered. Likewise, when probable and evaluative judgments are conflicting, communication and decision-making are much more difficult (see also Sparks and Turner, 2008).

Using PI theory as a framework for exploring how patients use information, we can see the interconnectedness between uncertainty and information as part of the decision-making process. As each patient and family member processes messages differently, health-care decision-making can be a complex communicative process.

The importance of information management in medical encounters

Patient participation in medical encounters is not a routine response action, but rather consists of the individual experience for each patient

(Eldh, Ekman, and Ehnfors, 2006). When we use information to empower ourselves in health-care interactions, sometimes the goal is to feel empowered by seeking information while at other times we feel empowered by a decision to avoid information about difficult health topics. A major part of patient empowerment consists in learning to harness the necessary time and energy to deal with health care. Barriers to patient empowerment can be both physical and emotional in nature.

Patient empowerment can be greatly influenced by the biological aspects of illness. For example, someone who is weak or dizzy may not feel motivated to engage in meaningful conversations with a doctor. Patients who physically feel sick may experience a sense of powerlessness in the treatment process, and may be less likely to take an active role in the medical encounter by openly expressing questions, concerns, and preferred treatment options. On the other hand, more interaction with a provider can empower someone in this situation, and can therefore create a greater sense of ownership over a disease or illness (McWilliam, Brown and Stewart, 2000).

In addition to the influence of a physical condition on communication, emotional influences may also lead to withdrawal from the social networks used to make sense of illness. Lack of communication with a provider can sometimes be the result of emotional drain, or even the need to deliberately conceal concerns that feel too threatening to be dealt with openly (Northouse and Northouse, 1988). In some cases, depression from chronic illness puts extreme strain on patients so communication in medical encounters is diminished (Dunkel-Schetter and Bennett, 1990). If a patient is willing and able to assert influence or agency in health-care interactions, this enables an active role in relating feelings to the provider, no matter how emotionally draining this process might be. Despite the physical and emotional challenges experienced by patients, there is significant evidence showing the importance of patient participation in medical encounters. Empowerment of patients can have a positive impact on healing because participating in decisions about health care, therapy, diet, and exercise can increase adherence to treatment regimens over time (Kenford and Fiore, 2004).

Other strategies for empowering patients to improve healing include meditation, relaxation, stress management techniques, expressing emotion, and "maintaining a sense of wonder about how the body will cooperate with medical treatment" (Kenford and Fiore, 2004). In other words, patients who actively participate in the care process become empowered partners in their own care. The empowered partner approach allows patients the opportunity to construct their own health-enabling lifestyle and maximizes the potential for self-care (McWilliam, 2009). Communication with providers about each of these opportunities can shift dialogue about what the patients cannot do, or what they must do, to what the patient can and should do to participate in the care process.

Health communication researcher Richard Street and colleagues have repeatedly demonstrated that patients are more likely to have positive health outcomes if they are actively involved in medical encounters (Street et al., 2005). Outcomes are also more positive when doctors are supportive and take the patient's perspective into consideration. Patient participation can be seen in many forms but there are specific behaviors that characterize active patient participation. Patient participation can occur through asking questions, expressing concerns and negative feelings, and being assertive. These are seen as active since they can lead to a powerful influence on the doctor's behavior and decision-making process (Street et al., 2003).

The majority of patients want precise information about their diagnosis and treatment options, and patients who participate in their overall decision-making often have better outcomes than patients who are not actively involved in this (Brown, et al., 2002; Pecchioni and Sparks, 2007; Sparks, 2007, forthcoming; Sparks and Turner, 2008). In fact, among patients aged 65 and older, nearly 85 percent of patients had better patient–provider relationships when they were well-informed about their prognosis (Repetto et al., 2009). Patients can be more proactive by seeking information from a variety of sources, including health-care organizations and the media, as well as being assertive regarding their health-care needs (Kahana and Kahana, 2003).

Patients understand that not all diagnoses are alike and not all patients are alike. For example, the interpretation of a diagnosis by a 20-year-old is often very different from that of a 90-year-old with the same diagnosis. These different interpretations are guided by varied life experiences, which can influence communication in the patient and provider relationship. Furthermore, it is important to understand that individuals of similar chronological age often undergo very different life experiences as well, and this also impacts interactions and perceptions in the patient and provider relationship (Sparks, 2007). One life experience that can dramatically differ for individuals of the same chronological age is the diagnosis of an advanced disease such as cancer (Sparks, 2007; Sparks and Turner, 2008). The impact of such a diagnosis, as well as subsequent interactions related to the diagnosis, can be overwhelming for older adult patients and those caring for them. Many older adults have experienced disease either themselves or through someone close to them, but more often these individuals have little experience with the unknown cancer culture and associated norms (Sparks, 2003a).

As patients enter the health-care environment, they must come with open ears and eyes as they embark upon a new cultural world of technical language; a sometimes unfriendly and stark atmosphere that can be very confusing and scary. Patients will not know all the answers, but each patient knows his or her symptoms and body better than any health-care provider. The important take-home message for patients is to "know thyself" and use that knowledge to communicate symptoms, feelings, hunches, and prior history. It is necessary to ask specific questions to get specific answers. Many providers will not understand or be familiar with each patient's cultural background or health beliefs, so patients have a responsibility to themselves to express key points as clearly as possible.

The relationship between physicians and patients plays a crucial role in patients' health outcomes (Street et al., 2003). Medical encounters have been characterized by control, role negotiation, health-care commitment, trust, and time and money issues (Walker et al., 2001). Overall, communication research in medical visits has concluded that about 66 percent of talk in these interactions is biomedically focused (Roter et al., 1997). Patients who desire two-way communication in health-care interactions still may not be willing to assume control, and some research indicates physicians are as much as six times more willing than patients to assume control of the encounter (von Friedrichs-Fitzwater and Gilgun, 2001). Physicians are typically able to achieve relational control of the medical encounter by focusing on the disease, changing topics, asking more questions, and talking more than the patient (ibid.).

Patient-centered communication (PCC) in medical encounters expands physician-patient communication from a physician-controlled biomedical information exchange to a relationship-building opportunity that integrates the medical examination with communication about social issues of the patient and family (von Friedrichs-Fitzwater and Gilgun, 2001). In 2001, the Institute of Medicine issued a call for the adoption of a PCC approach in medical encounters, and the Accreditation Council for Graduate Medical Education now requires competency in communication and relationship-building (Institute of Medicine, 2001; Accreditation Council for Graduate Medical Education, 1999).

Previous research has found that there are benefits to a patient-centered approach in medical encounters. First, PCC leads to patient involvement in the decision-making process (Beck, Daughtridge, and Sloan, 2002). Patients who report shared decision-making with their physician have more positive outcomes than patients who are not actively involved in the decision-making process (Brown et al., 2002), and patients who have high-quality contact with providers, including empathy on the latter's part, show reduction in pain and anxiety resulting from treatment (Dibbelt et al., 2009). PCC is associated with better recovery, better emotional health two months later, and fewer diagnostic tests and referrals (Stewart et al., 2000).

Second, PCC influences the patient's participation in medical encounters (Street et al., 2005). Findings also reveal that patients are more active when their physician engages in partnership-building and supportive talk (Street et al., 2005). Third, PCC contributes to relationship-building between physicians and patients. Patients' liking for their physician has been positively associated with better self-reported health, a more positive affective state after the visit, more favorable ratings of the physician's behavior, and greater visit satisfaction (Hall et al., 2002).

PCC research in medical encounters has been approached in a variety of ways. PCC has been conceptualized as the physician's understanding of the patient as a person, conveying empathy, finding common ground, and satisfaction (Swenson et al., 2004). Other elements of patient-centeredness, as reported by participants in the same study, include developing a good plan of care, listening, being open-minded, and taking into consideration the feelings of the patient. Still other studies have defined PCC as consisting of several variables including duration of medical encounter, physician's speech speed, physician's verbal dominance, ratio of patient-centered to physician-centered interviewing, positive patient affect and positive physician affect (Cooper et al., 2003). Despite all the research focus on what doctors can do to foster PCC, the point is that this approach is *patient-centered*. In other words, patients matter!

Brown, Stewart, and Ryan (2001) conceptualize PCC as being comprised of three dimensions: (1) exploring the disease and illness experience; (2) understanding the whole person; and (3) finding common ground.

Exploring the disease and illness experience

Communication about disease is embedded within the structure of the medical interview. Disease-specific information sharing allows the physician to identify abnormalities in the structure or function of the body wherein disease is the commonality that is shared with others (Brown et al., 2001). In contrast, illness is the patient's personal experience of ill health and it is unique to each individual (Brown et al., 2001). A patient-centered approach focuses on four dimensions of communication about illness: patient's feelings (e.g., fears about being ill); ideas about what is wrong with them; the effect of their problems on their function; and expectations about what should be done (Brown et al., 2001).

The physician must employ specific communicative strategies, such as open-ended questions, that allow the patient to express their concerns, rather than being limited to the short responses typically received from close-ended questions (Robinson and Heritage, 2006). Previous research has found that patients are more satisfied when physicians ask open-ended rather than close-ended questions (Robinson and Heritage, 2006). Further, barriers to treatment adherence can be better understood when providers ask open-ended questions to understand patients' concerns and assess change in the patients' attitudes (Hahn, 2009). Czaja et al. (2003) also discuss the importance of patient questions in the medical interaction and describe several important factors: the level of comfort a patient may feel about asking questions; the provider's clarity of answers; and the provider's response to information from other sources. All of these dimensions have a positive correlation with other forms of information-seeking behavior, such as using additional sources of information. Cegala et al. (2000) describe three types of questions present in physician–patient interviews. Direct questions are phrased in the standard form of a question. Assertive questions are actually declarative statements that serve information-seeking purposes. Indirect questions also have declarative phrasing, but lack apparent information-seeking qualities. Doctors may misinterpret patients' indirect questions as simple statements and not provide the desired information. Cegala et al. (2000) found that trained patients tended to ask more direct questions and received better answers from doctors. Thus, the research suggests that a patient's ability to ask questions and the level of comfort they feel about this, combined with the way in which a provider responds to outside information, affect a patient's information management behaviors.

Understanding the whole person

A physician's knowledge of a patient's family, work, beliefs, and struggles with life crises characterizes this second component of understanding the patient as a whole person in the context of their life setting (Brown, Stewart, and Ryan, 2001; Egbert et al., 2008; Sparks, 2003b, 2007). An earlier study of a doctor's communication style revealed several patterns that facilitate the inclusion of this type of information sharing (du Pré, 2001). The study found that the physician's self-disclosure of health and life experiences, expression of empathy, involvement of the patient in decision-making, open discussion of fears, the use of open-minded questions, and intent listening were successful techniques to enable and facilitate understanding of the whole person (du Pré, 2001).

According to Mishler (1984), physicians' talk tends to be characterized by the Voice of Medicine, which involves technical, medical jargon, whereas patients' talk resembles the Voice of the Lifeworld, reflecting both the social and cultural contexts of disease/illness. Active patient participation in medical encounters is characterized by communication behaviors such as asking questions, expressing concerns and negative feelings, and being assertive (Street et al., 2005). These behaviors are seen as active since they can lead to shared decision-making. An important aspect involves an understanding of the patients' religious views, especially with patients who are seriously ill. Patients cannot compartmentalize their lives, so illness must be viewed as a biological, psychological, and spiritual issue (Egbert et al., 2008; Geist-Martin, Sharf, and Jeha, 2008). Access to information, emotional needs, transportation availability, disruptions to work and family life, and financial burdens can all impact patient health and adherence to care (American Society of Clinical Oncology, 2009). Even though providers are most concerned with biological aspects of healing, patients must work to heal their bodies and their spirits during the care process. Spirituality is defined as "the search for what is sacred and holy in life" (Kliewer, 2004: 616) and includes topics directly related to illness, such as what happens after physical death, and what is the role of healing versus God's will for a patient.

Religion or spirituality may cause a struggle for patients who question the need for intervention by medical treatment on a plan put in place by God (Collins, Villagran, and Sparks, 2008). This fatalistic view of illness is common among some religions, and can make patient-centered medical decison-making very difficult for providers who are not sensitive to the issue. Patients may feel fatalistically powerless regarding their disease if they perceive it as a punishment from God, or part of God's plan for their life. Although this may be an uncomfortable area for some physicians (Geist-Martin et al., 2008), research suggests that patients who are able

to discuss their spiritual beliefs with their provider are more successful in making decisions about prevention and treatment, and more able
to cope with illness when it occurs (Kliewer, 2004; Geist-Martin et al.,
2008). However, empirical communication studies of this issue are lacking
(Egbert, Mickley, and Coeling, 2004).

Scholars generally agree that the terms "religiosity" and "spirituality" represent separate, although overlapping, concepts (Egbert et al.,
2008; Koenig, Larson, and McCullough, 2001; Paloutzian and Kirkpatrick,
1995; Parrott, 2004; Thoresen and Harris, 2002). Historically, religiosity has
received more scholarly attention than spirituality, especially in relation
to health outcomes (Parrott, 2004). In 1967, a classic work by Allport and
Ross differentiated between *intrinsic* religiosity, typically referring to living
according to one's religious beliefs because one truly believes in them and
extrinsic religiosity referring to using one's religion to meet needs such as
social support, tradition, or status. This differentiation has been maintained
by researchers for the past 40 years and has shaped our understanding of
how religion and religiosity are defined (Egbert et al., 2008).

Spirituality, on the other hand, is a more inclusive term, as it is considered to be a more expansive conceptualization of divinity. One may be a
spiritual person, but not necessarily religious; likewise, being a member
of a religion does not by definition make one spiritual (Egbert et al.,
2008). Whereas religion is associated with terms such as *formal, behavior-
oriented*, and *doctrine-based*, spirituality is better characterized using
words such as *individualistic, inward-directed, and not doctrine-oriented*
(Koenig et al., 2001). Although both are concepts worthy of discussions
related to their potential impact on the patient and provider relationship,
the central concept we wish to highlight here is found in the term *spirituality*, meaning an individual's search for meaning in life (e.g., Dreyer, 1994;
Egbert et al., 2008; National Cancer Institute, 2005). Along these lines, we
embrace Koenig et al.'s (2001) definition, "spirituality is the personal quest
for understanding answers to ultimate questions about life, about meaning, and about relationships to the sacred or transcendent, which may (or
may not) lead to or arise from the development of religious rituals and the
formation of community" (p. 18). Spirituality is an important element of an
individual's belief system, tending to impact health beliefs and decision-
making in patient and provider interaction. It is crucial that patients and
family members reveal such beliefs to their providers in an effort to achieve
higher-level understanding and to avoid miscommunication. By finding
common ground with their providers, patients can acquire more control of
their own health and treatment.

Finding common ground

Mutual undertaking to find common ground consists of physician–patient
communication and agreement about the nature of the problem, the goals
of treatment and management, and the roles of the patient and physician
(Brown, Stewart, and Ryan, 2001). Du Pré (2001) suggests that the process

of informed consent about treatment risks, benefits, and options is one way for physicians and patients to reach a common understanding.

An absence of PCC can lead to less information sharing, miscommunication, and misunderstandings. Miscommunication between patients and providers can have serious consequences, especially when the information is related to a patient's diagnosis or treatment plan. Health-related information is often presented at a level above the patients' reading ability. When providers use technical scientific language to describe a patient's diagnosis, to avoid embarrassment the patient may not admit his or her lack of understanding. Egbert et al. (2008) suggest considering how some of the more complex terms used by physicians could be simplified to increase patients' understanding of the information.

Patients can be encouraged to participate through allowing them to share personal stories that provide important cues regarding their attitudes and beliefs toward illness, medicine, and health behaviors (Young and Rodriguez, 2006). When a provider can take the time to focus and listen closely to patients' stories it can give important insight into specific values, the mental constructs that drive patients' decision-making, and the goals for the medical visit. Patient participation is enhanced because the stories told create an opportunity for sharing, and a basis for two-way communication.

There is some question as to whether *all* patients want to be active participants in their own health care. Evidence suggests there may be cultural and generational differences that can predict which patients are more comfortable with a traditional relationship (where the doctor is seen as the authority figure) and which patients prefer to be in charge of their own health-care decisions (and view the physician as a consultant or an advisor). *Concordance* is defined as a shared similarity, or shared identity, between physician and patient, based on a demographic attribute such as race, sex, or age (Street et al., 2008). When patients perceive similarity between themselves and their provider, they are more likely to be satisfied with their health-care experience and trust their provider, with adherence to their treatment over time (Street et al., 2008).

In other words, concordance is the extent to which a patient sees a provider as being similar enough to him or her to trust the provider and follow treatment recommendations. For example, a female might feel more comfortable telling a female Ob/Gyn about her menstrual cramps. However, if the Ob/Gyn is a male, there is less certainty that he can empathize with with the problem. That could lead to less active participation or satisfaction with the relationship.

Some researchers have found that a patient's desire to be involved in their health care may vary, based on educational and generational differences (Clark et al., 2009), because older patients are likely to prefer a traditional model of listening and following orders, versus sharing in conversation and decisions. One challenge for increased patient participation is that some patients, such as older adults, often seek a direct style from their doctors (Eldh, Ekman, and Ehnfors, 2006). To overcome this and encourage interaction, providers can use communication tools such as written questionnaires, patient checklists, or a diary to elicit participation by timid patients (Klingenberg et al., 2005).

Street et al. (2003, 2005) suggest that a healthy balance between authority and consultation creates better communication and partnership-building. In fact, patients who share control of the medical encounter tend to be more interactive with providers and the mutual influence creates a good balance of communication. To participate effectively in medical encounters, patients have to believe that their opinions matter, and that there is value in shared decision-making processes (Street, 2007). If the provider is the pilot, the patient can still buy a ticket to their preferred destination! In other words, we may not be able to fully dictate the course of our health care, but we can and should value the communication process between providers and patients as a vital part of our health care.

In addition to improving partnership-building and shared decision-making, the Joint Commission on Accreditation of Healthcare Organizations (JCAHO) encourages patients to engage in communication with providers to help prevent medical errors. JCAHO promotes a program entitled SPEAK UP as a way to educate and empower patients to become active, involved, and informed about their care. SPEAK UP is an acronym that conveys the following ideas.

S: Speaking up means asking the right questions and expecting to receive answers that you can understand. If you are not comfortable with the words used by a provider, ask them to clarify what is said using more non-technical, non-scientific language.

P: Pay attention to the care you are receiving. Patients can be their own watchdog to make sure you are getting the right medication and the right treatment. As a patient you should communicate your concern if you notice inconsistencies. Watch for simple things like making sure your pills look the same each time your prescription is filled, or watching to be sure health-care providers wash their hands or use clean gloves when examining you.

E: Educate yourself about your diagnosis, tests, and treatment. Being an informed consumer of health information occurs through active participation in your own health care. For example, if you write down notes as your doctor talks to you about your condition, you can use them later to gather information from a variety of sources to make sense of your illness. Reading forms before you sign them can provide you with important information about side-effects, treatment options, and potential negative outcomes associated with your illness. Doctors do not always verbally tell patients everything about their illness, and patients have both the right and the responsibility to be savvy consumers of information. Educating yourself makes you more able to ask the right questions, and make choices that are right for you and your family.

A: Ask a family member or friend to accompany you on your doctor visits. Communication with a doctor can be difficult if you are sick or worried, so having a companion along can give you an advocate to ask questions, or listen to information you might need to recall later.

K: Know exactly which pills you take, and why you take them. This can be especially challenging when you are ill, or if you have to take several different pills at differing intervals during the day. Some people use special pill boxes to keep track of their medication, and some people use an alarm or buzzer to remind them to take a treatment. Communicate with your family or roommates about your treatment plan and medication, then they can help you by noticing inconsistencies, and by understanding the importance of not moving or rearranging your pills in the cabinet.

U: Use health-care facilities that are accredited and clean. While it may be tempting to get a tattoo or piercing in a backroom of a bar in Tijuana, it is neither safe nor smart. Communicate with providers to inquire about their safety record, and their procedures for after-care once you are discharged. Some medical facilities have a published safety record that you can find on the Internet, or get from your local or state government. The main idea is to use your best judgment about health care because the people and place where you receive it should look (and be) healthy.

P: Participate in your own care because you are the most important member of your health-care team. Patient participation occurs through active information management and open communication with providers.

Be honest, and (at least try to) have fun!

Patients who perceive their provider to be significantly more powerful than themselves may not be completely honest about certain habits, risky behaviors, or lack of adherence to a medical treatment plan. Perceived power differences can influence adult patients to feel more like adolescents who conceal certain behaviors from their parents and teachers. The problem with withholding important information from providers is that patients who deceive their providers on routine questions about alcohol consumption, sexual activity, or diet only hurt themselves by painting an inaccurate picture of their own health. Patients might think it is embarrassing or uncomfortable to admit to engaging in unprotected sex or binge drinking, but the reality is that doctors ask questions because they use the information provided in the answers to make diagnoses and recommendations, and to avoid medical errors. Deceiving doctors because it is difficult to be honest about risky behavior opens the door for ineffective or dangerous medical decision-making.

Ways to avoid deception

Work closely with your doctor.

- Open communication with your doctor is absolutely crucial throughout the health-care process. Your doctor will be asking for your feedback on treatment protocols and medication side-effects, so pay attention to how you are responding to your treatment.

- Don't hold back on sharing any symptoms, questions, or concerns because every piece of information is important. The more your doctor knows, the better he or she can help you.

Open communication with a provider means patients should always:

- *Tell your doctor about other medical conditions.*
- You and your doctor have probably already discussed your medical history and other conditions you may have. However, if you're unsure that your doctor has all your medical information, talk with him or her openly and honestly about any existing conditions you currently have.
- *Discuss any medications you are taking for other conditions.*
- You and your doctor have probably also discussed medications or other types of treatments you are taking for other conditions. If you do not share all information about your current medications, or if you forget to include over-the-counter medicine or herbal remedies, inform your doctor right away. Remember, complete honesty with your provider helps build your relationship and improves your care over time.

To overcome difficulties in communicating problematic topics in medical encounters, some research indicates that the use of humor by patients and providers can reduce perceptions of power differences and promote healthier medical relationships. Research on humor in medical interviews supports the importance of gender roles and professional roles as a source of power in medical interviews, and even suggests that patients of female doctors are more likely to use humor than patients of male doctors (Sala, Krupat, and Roter, 2002).

Obviously, a doctor who uses inappropriate humor will only make an uncomfortable situation even worse. Imagine for example, a doctor kidding about STD, or making a patient believe he or she has an incurable disease rather than just a cold – inappropriate humor is never funny! Appropriate humor, however, can reduce a patient's apprehension about sharing personal information, and can alleviate fears about perceived disapproval by doctors (Scholl, 2007). Humor can help ease the tension and lighten the mood of a medical interview. Used well, it can help establish rapport that enhances information sharing and makes patients feel more at ease. Patients who use humor may also exhibit a more positive attitude, and may also be happier in general (Scholl and Ragan, 2003).

Functions of affect in medical encounters

> Patients and their loved ones swim together with physicians in a sea of feelings. Each needs to keep an eye on a neutral shore where flags are planted to warn of perilous emotional currents.
>
> Groopman, 2007: 58

One of the common themes of this chapter is that not only the thoughts of patients, but their feelings, impact the way they think about their providers, health-care options, and the decisions they make in health-care interactions (Sparks and Turner, 2008). Emotion, or affect, can be a mood we have before we arrive at a medical encounter, or it can be triggered by our experiences, memories, or perceptions of illness. Certain words can trigger emotion that clouds our judgment, or prevents us from focusing on the conversation. If a provider casually mentions the "C" word (cancer) a few months after the patient's mother just died of cancer, the patient might have a much stronger reaction than if s/he had no experience with the disease (Sparks, 2003b). Words trigger emotions, and emotion can either get in the way of making clear decisions or it can factor into the decision itself. If a cancer patient cannot emotionally handle the thought of losing all her hair from chemotherapy, she will be reluctant to choose chemotherapy treatment if there is another option (Sparks and Villagran, 2008). The ways in which individuals cognitively process health messages vary, but can be greatly impacted by emotion or affect (Sparks, 2007; Sparks and Turner, 2008). Patients will make health decisions before, during, and after each medical encounter with their providers. As such, it is important for patients and providers to have a basic understanding of the underpinnings of cognitive processing and the impact of affect on processing.

According to the heuristic systematic model (Chaiken, 1980) and the theoretically similar elaboration likelihood model (ELM), people will process messages via systematic processing, heuristic processing, or both. When a patient processes a health message heuristically, s/he typically considers few message cues, and instead forms his/her judgment based on simple decision-making. For instance, the patient may read a website encouraging meditation as a therapy for cancer. The content may (or may not) have been written by a medical doctor. Thus, the patient may believe the website, thinking that "medical doctors can be trusted," instead of critically thinking about (and cross-checking) the message. Other simple cues may be "longer messages are better," "doctors are more trustworthy," "all my friends are doing it," or "physically attractive people are more likeable." People processing in this mode do not differentiate between weak and strong health messages, but rather are persuaded by variables irrelevant to message processing (Chaiken, 1980; Petty and Cacioppo, 1986; Petty, Cacioppo, and Goldman, 1981). This kind of processing can be dangerous in the realm of the medical communication encounter where misinformation can lead to poor prevention practices, or an inability to detect a serious disease.

Patients who process messages systematically will think carefully about the health message and engage in thinking relevant to the message content (see, e.g., Sparks, 2007; Sparks and Turner, 2008). Individuals, however, are economical and will invest only the necessary cognitive effort to complete the task at hand. And, in order to engage in systematic processing, people must be sufficiently motivated and have sufficient cognitive resources. Motivation is affected by how personally relevant the message is (Chaiken, 1980), the reader's need for cognition (Cacioppo et al., 1986), exposure to unexpected message contents (Maheswaran and Chaiken, 1991), and, in many cases, the number of messages received. Cognitive resources, or ability to process a message, are affected by distraction (Festinger and Maccoby, 1964; Petty, Wells, and Brock, 1976), message repetition (Cacioppo and Petty, 1979), time pressure (Moore, Hauskneckt, and Thamodaran, 1986), communication modality (Eagly and Chaiken, 1993), and knowledge and expertise (Alba and Marmorstein, 1987).

Attitude change that occurs due to systematic processing is more durable, and indicative of future behavior change. This is because such attitudes were formed by careful evaluation of the merits of the arguments and, thus, reflect the content of the thoughts that were generated while reading (or listening to) the message. If these arguments are perceived to be high quality, the message receiver should generate positive thoughts. But if the message is viewed as low quality, the thoughts generated by the message will be negative, leading to less persuasion. In this way, systematic processing is what Sparks and Turner (2008) call the "holy grail" of cognitive processing. It is believed that if we can motivate careful processing, message receivers will engage in message elaboration and convince themselves to engage in the recommended actions. Further, they are more likely to engage in long-term change. For patients, this may mean the difference between detecting a serious disease such as cancer and living, or failing to detect cancer and dying.

Systematic processing is manifested in various ways. Cognitive processes refer to such information-processing activities as perceiving, abstracting, judging, elaborating, rehearsing, and recalling from memory. The most common method of examining cognitive responses in research is to ask participants to list or report all of their thoughts after having read (or heard) a message. These messages can be mass mediated or interpersonal in nature. Categorically, these thoughts can be counter-arguments, favorable thoughts, or irrelevant thoughts. And it should be noted that these thoughts can relate to the message, the source, the audience of the message, or the channel through which the message was transmitted (Cacioppo, Harkins, and Petty, 1981).

Positive thoughts reflect relative agreement with the message. If such thoughts occur after having read a message carefully, these positive cognitions will be predictive of long-term change. That is, when positive thoughts occur because people have carefully considered the merits of an appeal, have cross-checked that message, and/or have researched the issue themselves, then the likelihood that they will actually engage in the actions recommended in the message is high. Yet people can have positive thoughts after barely attending to a message, or after having heuristically processed a message. Therefore, it is important to also look at where the positive thoughts were directed. Positive thoughts about the source (the source is a likeable person; the source is an expert) may reveal a lack of careful thinking (Sparks, 2007; Sparks and Turner, 2008).

Counter-arguments are negative thoughts regarding the persuasive message where the message receiver counters an argument in the message. The more counter-arguments people generate after having received a message, the less likely they are to be motivated to engage in the actions recommended in the message (Sparks and Turner, 2008). Thus, when listening to such prevention and detection messages, patients must be aware of the potential processing pitfalls that can easily impact sound decision-making. Several factors are known to increase counter-arguing. If a patient is motivated to form an unfavorable opinion (e.g., if s/he is cynical about colorectal cancer exams), careful thought can take the form of arguing against the message (Petty, Wells, and Brock, 1976). Also, if a person has an unbalanced amount of information about the message topic, they may be more biased when processing the message (Petty and Wegener, 1999). Counter-arguing is decreased as the message arguments increase in quality. Thus, the more well-thought out the arguments, the more the source of the message understands the arguments against the recommendations (e.g., the side-effects of treatment), the more statistical and narrative evidence that can be provided, the less likely the patient (or provider) will counter-argue. It must be noted, however, that counter-arguing is also decreased when people are distracted (Buller, 1986) or when people are in a good mood (Janis, Kaye, and Kirschner, 1965), indicating that decreased counter-arguing is not always a good thing. Instead, we must all recognize why patients (or providers) have reduced counter-argumentation.

Message receivers can also have irrelevant thoughts when receiving a health message (Sparks and Turner, 2008). In such cases, the message receiver thinks about entirely different issues when receiving a message. Irrelevant thoughts can take the form of "I was thinking about grocery shopping while my doctor was talking to me," or "I am afraid of dying so I turned my thoughts to something more positive." Especially in patient–provider communication where the topic is likely to conjure up thoughts of death, fear, or even recollections of the loss of a loved one, message designers must take into consideration how to keep thoughts on task (Sparks, 2003b). Importantly, health communication and persuasion researchers have acknowledged the importance of designing persuasive messages to induce motivation in receivers to increase the likelihood of systematic processing (Sparks, 2007; Sparks and Turner, 2008). We must tackle these unknowns in order to develop better, clearer, more effective communication in the patient and provider relationship.

There are four functions of emotion in health communication: affect as information, affect as spotlight, affect as a motivator, and affect as common currency (Peters, Lipkus, and Defenbach, 2006). Affect as information refers to how patients make decisions based on their sense of how two alternatives feel compared to one another. Deciding to engage in a risky health behavior such as binge drinking might feel good at the time, but how will it feel the day after? That information might impact decisions to drink or not to drink in the future.

Affect as spotlight means that how a person feels about a certain health issue impacts the way it is talked about with a provider. A patient might focus on a certain aspect of a problem because it seems the most important to him or her, such as asking a provider if it is true people gain weight when they quit smoking instead of asking about the long-term benefits of such a choice. Weight gain is the highlighted piece of information because it is the most worrying.

Affect as motivator refers to the tremendous power of emotion to motivate or deter action. For example, a young woman named Zahara explained in her online journal that she is afraid to find out what will happen to her brain if she tries Ecstasy, so she never takes the drug when her friends do. She is just too scared. Fear can motivate a person to go get a flu shot, stay away from tobacco, or take time to read up on the causes of diabetes. We seek out ways to combat our fear because we are motivated to do so by our emotional response to an issue or problem.

The final function of affect is as a common currency (Peters et al., 2006). When we think about health-related decisions, we often weigh the costs and benefits of two alternatives. We don't just think about the information itself, but rather we compare how we feel about alternative A versus alternative B. Even when two options are very different, what makes it easier for us to choose when presented with alternatives by our doctor is that we focus on the affect associated with both options. Information can be confusing and complex, but we all can understand fear, or sadness, or joy. Another online journal by a teenager named David described how great his relationships were when he took his anti-depression medication, so the decision to stick with his treatment was much easier because he was experiencing true friendships for the first time. He compared his satisfaction with life while he was on medication versus his life when he was off medication, and it was very simple to decide that he would take his pills regularly.

Conclusion

Medical decision-making is, at its very core, a communicative act. We seek or avoid information to help us gain a sense of control, or at least participation in the care process. The extent to which we can truly make decisions about our health care lies in the nature and severity of illness. In this chapter we have examined the importance of information for patients who seek to take part in their own medical decision-making, and we have looked at barriers to open communication with providers. Medical encounters are not usually fun or easy, but most doctors want to make the process as comfortable for patients as possible. When there is an opportunity to lighten the moment with a humorous comment, or share an emotional concern, doctors and patients can connect with each other by asking good questions, giving honest answers, and working together to find the best medical solutions for the patient. Patients who engage in shared decisions are more likely to be satisfied with their doctor, and often have better health outcomes, so it is worth taking the time to prepare with information and questions perceived as important, based on the situation, before each visit to a doctor.

Discussion Questions for Patients to ask Providers

Communication with a health-care provider is essential to improving care and ensuring that a patient achieves desired health outcomes. While providers are responsible for giving accurate and useful health information, it is also important for a patient to ask questions. Coming to the office prepared with questions can help to alleviate stress and to open communication. The following questions are a good starting point for facilitating conversation with a provider.

How long have you been practicing medicine?

Where did you go to school and what kind of training do you have that is related to my illness?

Can you describe my treatment method in detail? What are the side-effects I might experience? What types of changes do I need to make in my personal life during treatment?

How should I expect to feel during my treatment?

How much will treatment cost?

Have you treated other patients with the same problem? Could I speak with any of them?

What type of special supplies might I need during treatment? Where can I get these supplies?

How long will it be before we know if treatment is working or not?

What is the best-case scenario for the outcome of my treatment? What are my odds of achieving that outcome?

How might treatment affect my sex life? Are there ways to maintain intimacy with my partner that I can use during treatment?

I'm feeling stressed. How have others coped with the emotional roller-coaster of treatment?

4 Provider Characteristics

Narrative from Kristin (not her real name):

Sometimes it seems my whole life has revolved around depression. When I was only four, the birth of my brother brought my mother the gift of postpartum depression. To this day, 19 years later, I can still remember my mom sleeping entire days away while my dad and I took care of my brother and sister. Life changes, and with it, so do one's capabilities to handle these changes. After I graduated from college and moved, suddenly I was very introverted. I knew I wasn't extremely depressed, but I wasn't handling anxiety well at all. I was trying to control everything, while I knew on some level this was not possible. Because I knew depression and its symptoms so well, I decided to finally see a doctor. I knew my problems couldn't be helped by a psychologist because mostly I was upset about what the future would bring. I decided, through talks with my mother and friends, that the best plan would be to try medication. I can still remember nervously making the appointment.

Because my entire family suffers from a form of mental illness, I figured it would not be hard to talk to the doctor. Surely he would see that I knew how I was feeling, and would listen when I said what medication I wanted. I was wrong. When the doctor came in, I suddenly became very nervous about spilling my mental problems with him. While I knew he was a doctor, no one ever wants to seem "crazy." I did try my best though to explain how I was feeling and what I wanted to feel again. He heard me, but he didn't listen to me. As soon as I was done talking, he suggested I take a depression test before he would write a prescription. I agreed, because it was the only way to get what I wanted. This test was a complete joke. There were 30 questions which all required an answer ranging from "never" to "most of the time," and the questions asked things like, do you feel "down in the dumps?" It was obvious to me that most of these didn't apply to my situation because I told the doctor I was anxious, not depressed. So I answered the questions to the best of my ability, knowing full well what my answers were going to reveal to the doctor. As I sat there on the examination table, I wondered how this test could ever be considered valid. If someone was coming in to prove to a loved one they weren't depressed, they could just answer "never" to each question. If someone was coming in to get medication, like myself, they could answer just enough to warrant the meds. Eventually a nurse came in to take my test from me and after about 15 minutes the doctor came in with my results. I was only marginally depressed. This news didn't shock me at all. He said he was going to prescribe medication that would help with the anxiety, but he never told me what the medication was. After that revelation, he walked out and a nurse delivered my prescription for this mystery medication. It was Zoloft, the one med I did not want. I knew many people who had taken this drug only to gain a good amount of weight, lose all of their sexual appetite, and actually have more suicidal tendencies. I was astounded the doctor prescribed it to me, a 23-year-old female. I left the doctor feeling scared and only a little hopeful.

I took the Zoloft for about two months and gained 20 pounds. Not only that, I felt like it wasn't working. I decided to see another doctor and this time I decided to directly tell the doctor the name of the medication I would like to try to see what he thought. After my visit with this doctor I felt he never questioned my understanding of my own feelings, and I felt he trusted my judgment of my own situation. I left with a new prescription for Wellbutrin and a better sense of control. I learned that even though there is a stigma attached to mental illness, you have to take matters into your own hands. Doctors can't help you unless you help them understand you by communicating your needs.

Anonymous

In this chapter, we explore the art and science of the medical encounter from the providers' perspective. While the previous chapter focused on the information needs of patients, this chapter takes a closer look at the verbal and non-verbal strategies employed by providers when interacting with patients and their families. In addition, listening, empathy, and consequences of miscommunication and poor communication are explored.

Physicians are the primary and most influential sources of information, with supplemental information from other health-care providers, informal social networks, and information outlets such as the Internet. Research from the NCI 2005 Health Information National Trends Survey indicates that when participants were asked "Where would you go for cancer information," 50 percent stated they would go to their provider, followed by Internet (34 percent), library (5 percent), family (4 percent), and print media (4 percent). In fact, recent research supporting the NCI study indicated that the only source of health information that older adults use consistently is their doctor (Pecchioni and Sparks, 2007).

The authors further found that after doctors, the most important information sources were (in order): family members, nurses, friends, the Internet, other medical personnel, and other patients. However, the source of information that patients were most satisfied with was their friends and family. The source of information they were least satisfied with was listed as their doctor. These data indicate a serious discrepancy between information sought and information that people are satisfied with (Pecchioni and Sparks, 2007). This is a critical issue for health practitioners because information provided by friends and family may lack up-to-date research, clarity, or even accuracy. For example, friends and family members might talk about a series of vaccines or a chemotherapy regimen they had 10 or 15 years ago as the way things are done. In reality, medical protocols are constantly evolving and becoming more efficient. Thus, there is often a mythology that pervades people's understandings of disease and treatment, especially cancer. Further, physician behavior has been found to impact medical adherence and decision-making (Tinley et al., 2004).

Physicians have a difficult time delivering all of the crucial health-care information that may be needed by patients and generally do not tailor their delivery of information to the knowledge levels of their patients (Pecchioni and Sparks, 2007; Sparks and Turner, 2008). Time constraints, competing demands for attention, and a lack of training in effective communication impair physicians' delivery of comprehensive information to patients, particularly when it comes to bad news delivery (Pecchioni and Sparks, 2007; Sparks et al., 2007). Health-care providers are accustomed to processing highly complex medical information while their patients are typically less familiar with this.

One of the basic skills a health-care provider must learn is how to conduct a medical interview (Beck, Daughtridge, and Sloan, 2002). This interview forms the basis for all diagnosis and treatment of an illness. A successful and communicative medical interview helps inform patients about important information related to the diagnosis or treatment plan, and can lead to more patient involvement in the decision-making process (Sparks, Travis, and Thompson, 2005). Providers who successfully engage patients in thinking through options and making decisions regarding their treatment have more positive outcomes than those experienced when patients simply follow orders without being actively involved (Brown et al., 2002). The process of the medical interview is the essential structure through which health care first occurs, and it sets the stage for a patient's perception of health and illness, future health-care interactions, treatment adherence, and shared decision-making. Skilled providers, whether formal (e.g., doctors, nurses) or informal (family caregivers), can listen for the subtle communicative cues such as humor, self-disclosure, or narratives that naturally arise during interaction with patients (Sparks, Travis, and Thompson, 2005).

Often, a patient's words and gestures are composed of ambiguous signals, and require interpretation (Sillars et al., 2000). Bateson (1972) was one of the first theorists to note that communication involves more than simple message translation. The interviewer and interviewee communicate with each other and also communicate about the communication. Each interactant in a conversation plants cues (humorous anecdotes, for example) to suggest how a message should be handled. Adding to the complexity of the puzzle, the participants themselves are often unaware of the cues they are sending and may effortlessly attend to and present cues in their talk (duPré, 1998). What this means for health and human service professionals is that the way they were taught to conduct interviews in their educational programs is probably not adequate for the complex interview situations they will find in many settings today.

As Sparks et al. (2005) describe, long-term family caregivers are frequently asked to talk about topics such as bowel movements, loneliness, personal safety, and intimate care. Such socially taboo and sensitive topics can cause periods of awkwardness and embarrassment. When caregivers must share this information with others, and in the process expose their own personal fears and shortcomings about their caregiving abilities, humorous anecdotes and laughter can help caregivers manage a multitude of face-threatening situations. To fully appreciate the subtlety and complexity of this communication strategy it is important to understand that the humorous anecdote is not the end point. Rather, humor is the cue that sensitive probing may now be in order to fully understand what the caregiver is experiencing, feeling, and shadowing from the interviewer (Sparks, Travis, and Thompson, 2005).

Social workers, physicians, nurses, and other health and human services providers conduct numerous "interviews" and historical accounts of their patients' lives, yet often fail to probe for deeper and richer information that may be just beyond the "typical" interview exchange. How can interviewers (providers) make the most of the short time spent with patients and loved ones in an information-gathering conversation? How can interviewers better understand the communicative cues that patients and their loved ones are using to "convey meaning" about their personal situations to the listener?

These principles are especially important when difficult subjects, such as breaking bad news, are involved (Buckman et al., 1997; Gillotti, Thompson, and McNeilis, 2002; Sparks et al., 2007). Only by listening to the client and his or her family can professionals truly understand the implications of the illness, problem, or need for the client and family (Buckman, et al., 1997; du Pré and Beck, 1997).

Health and human service providers spend from 45 to 70 percent of their time every day listening to others (Johnson, 1996). The ability of these professionals to listen carefully is directly linked to their ability to recognize what is important in the conversation (Canary, Cody, and Manusov, 2000). For instance, in the case of long-term family caregivers, there appears to be a heavy reliance on the communicative use of humor to convey information about caregiving issues and the condition of the care recipient (Sparks-Bethea et al., 2000). While most health and human service professionals have been taught interviewing and active-listening techniques to enable the speaker to clarify a message (Cooper, 1995; Johnson, 1996), they may not readily apply the humor as an important part of these conversations.

In addition to their professional knowledge and experience, doctors possess personal characteristics, values, biases, and skills that impact every medical interaction. Although many of us as patients feel it is most important for a physician to be knowledgeable, we also need to obtain information from our provider, and ideally to feel that the person in charge of our health program really cares about who we are as people too (Tait, 2007).

Based on these ideas, in some ways the medical interview is similar to the first day of a college course for patients and providers. Obviously, the expectations for a doctor visit are very different from those for a college course, but the outcome is very similar. The patient is like the student who goes to the first day of class to gather information. Like health care, college is expensive so patients and students do their homework to select classes and doctors who can help fulfill a need. Sometimes we use the Internet to gather information, and sometimes we talk to friends and family to make our selection of a class or a provider who we feel is the best "match" between our personal preferences and the choices available. In school we seek out the professor who teaches the right class at the right time, and preferably has a great reputation on campus. In health care we seek out the doctor who has the right location and specialty, who participates in a particular insurance plan, and preferably who has a great reputation in the community.

The goal of the first medical visit and the first day of class is to get information about what to expect next, but there is certainly a personal dimension to both situations as well. Does a person trust the doctor/professor's word? Does s/he sound like s/he knows the subject matter well? Does someone feel comfortable enough to continue with this relationship? If not, is it too late to drop the class, or to find another doctor to get a second opinion? We like to engage with doctors and professors whom we feel are knowledgeable, trustworthy, and personable. This is not always possible, based on constraints of the system in which we are operating, but we certainly make judgments about the person with whom we are interacting. Doctors and professors are both in positions of power, so we want to be sure they will earn that power, and not take advantage of it. Depending on how flexible we can be with all our preferences, we may or may not choose to look elsewhere if we don't find what we are looking for on the first try. Sometimes, however, it is a relief just to get health care or a class, so we make the decision to stick with the doctor or professor, regardless of our first impressions.

Once a provider is selected, we expect to gain something from our visit, so to accomplish our goals we typically expect providers to be highly skilled at maintaining professional, productive, and practiced conversations with patients and their families. Despite great advances in the development of new protocols and drugs to diagnose and treat patients, communication between providers and patients remains one of the most cost-effective means of improving medical outcomes. First impressions count. Providers who give their patients undivided attention for the first 60 seconds of the medical encounter are more likely to leave their patients feeling satisfied with care than those who seem distracted or disinterested (Rea, 2010).

It is not unusual for a physician to engage in upwards of 150,000 medical encounters during his or her working lifetime (Eggly, 2002). It is vitally important that physicians learn to listen to and support the needs of their patients. In an effort to adequately prepare for a career filled with medical interviews with patients bringing a plethora of medical, social, and cultural issues, many providers develop their own theories concerning proper and accepted communication with patients (Groopman, 2007). The steps of the health-care process are charted over and over, each time a new patient comes in with a new set of symptoms. Health-care providers' thought processes are guided by a set of routine questions. What is the problem today? What is your medical history? Does it hurt when I push here?

When a patient comes in to the office with a medical concern, the major goal of the interaction becomes diagnosis (Tait, 2007). Diagnosis is both an end and a beginning in the treatment process and until the point when the diagnosis is made, the provider and patient have to work together through their interaction to share information that will facilitate a proper diagnosis. After the diagnosis is reached, the communication between physician and patient must turn to discussions related to "what do we do now?" The interaction between physician and patient in the context of a proper treatment schedule should be shaped by characteristics of the patient, but often characteristics of the provider create the lens through which the interaction is viewed.

Success in involving a patient in the implementation and progression of a treatment plan is markedly influenced by the physician's communication style and ability. Physician communication has been described in terms of the content (i.e., cost and benefits of specific recommendations for treatment, medication, etc.), as well as relational factors that may lend themselves to the use of a particular style, such as enthusiasm or immediacy (Kahana and Kahana, 2007; Query and Kreps, 1996). Additional factors likely to affect this communication style may include simple things such as where he or she was born and raised, and the attitudes, values, and beliefs taken from his/her background; educational experience; the provider's own physical and emotional state; self-esteem level; commitment level to *this* patient and the outcome of the treatment; and feedback from the patient (Tait, 2007).

Many women and a growing number of men will choose a female physician because they may feel that she will be "more understanding." For example, female physicians tend to use more positive talk, may ask more questions, perhaps suggest counseling more freely, and may seem more emotionally focused during the interview (Roter, Hall and Aoki, 2002). There seems to be little to no difference between male and female doctors in the amount or quality of scientific information provided, but more personal inquiries made by female physicians may result in longer and more satisfying interviews (Roter et al., 2002). Gender is one example of how provider characteristics can shape their general approach to the medical encounter. Ideally, each medical interview is unique, but in reality providers often slide into a comfort zone of rehearsed steps used in each encounter with a patient regardless of the unique qualities possessed by a particular patient or situation. There is a tendency for the process of a medical interview to become routine and systematic, but effectively "reaching" a patient to interact with him or her can be much more difficult (Bronfin, 2008). Robinson and Heritage (2006) note that the medical interview is generally organized in six different phases: opening, problem presentation, information gathering, diagnosis, treatment, and closing. A physician may feel that, other than the presentation of the problem, the remainder of the interview should be conducted solely by the physician, and may become annoyed when a patient interrupts the routine (Robinson and Heritage, 2006). Many doctors prefer to interrupt or redirect a patient's remarks or answers to questions and move them back to the safe and satisfying routine previously constructed for an interview. This tendency leads to strictly one-sided interactions that can be almost totally void of input from the patient. Physicians sometimes even interrupt patients when the patient is answering the doctor's question (Koehn et al., 2007).

Physician–patient communication tends to be asymmetrical because doctors often exert more control than patients over the style and content of the interaction (Koehn et al., 2007). Physicians give information, ask closed-ended questions, talk about the meaning of symptoms, discuss treatment options, and give patients instructions in a way that allows the provider to maintain control of the conversation. When providers seem determined to maintain control of the path of conversation in medical interactions, they can utilize predictable scripts for generating patient responses and moving through the steps of the interview without really engaging with the patient at all.

Perhaps providers dominate communication because of time constraints, or because answers to their questions provide data that will be used to diagnose potential problems, order tests, or refer the patient to specialists. When the provider fails to engage in active listening and communication with a patient, medical mistakes are likely to occur and opportunities are lost for improved patient outcomes. In fact, research indicates that 80 percent of medical errors are due to communication breakdown (JCAHO, 2002).

This situation is similar to the drive home after a long, hard day. Someone who has worked in a job for more than five years may know the route by heart. There are no major traffic accidents; no bad weather along the way. It is just a routine drive. From getting in the car, listening to favorite music on an iPod, a person may next be aware of pulling in the driveway without remembering details of the journey as if having been in autopilot to get home. A neighbor may come a moment after you arrive and say, "Hey, I was waving and honking at you on the way home, but you didn't notice."

People have an existing mental map, or schema, that help them navigate the path from office to home, sometimes actively engaging with other cars or people on the way, and sometimes not. Many health-care providers are the same. They have schema that they have developed as a result of many patient interactions, many tests ordered and read, and many meetings with their health-care team. The mental map eliminates the need for real connection or real interaction with the patient.

Historical evolution of providers in medical encounters

The evolution of the doctor–patient relationship has been the focus of significant research. Rutten and Arora (2007) outline three distinct models of provider–patient communication. The first model, the *biomedical* or *paternalistic* approach to patient care was popular in the 1950s and 1960s.

In this model, physicians were almost always seen as authority figures, and patients were most typically compliant (Parsons, 1951; Steinhart, 2002). The second approach is called the *consumeristic* model, where doctors are a source of information for health-care consumers who have autonomy in making decisions about their care. Consumerism in health care implies that well-informed patients are best equipped to decide among treatment options, and that control over decisions should lie solely with the patient (Emanual and Emanual, 1992; Rutten and Arora, 2007). A third, more contemporary, model of health care is the shared decision-making model. In this approach, patients and providers work together to exchange information and ideas, and collaboratively create each medical encounter. This approach has been called the *relationship-centered model* (Rutten and Arora, 2007), and closely resembles Epstein and Street's (2007) conception of patient-centered communication. In recent decades, providers have begun to consider the benefits of shared patient decision-making and many have turned to patient-centered approaches to care (see chapter 4). Despite this trend, in a 2000 Kaiser Family Foundation survey of 2,000 adults (American Society for Quality, February 2005, p. 15), 4 in 10 persons reported the quality of health care had deteriorated in the last five years; 4 in 10 believed it had remained about the same; and just 1 in 10 indicated that quality had improved. There is no question that the health-care system is strained, so providers and patients must make the most of each encounter. The importance of relational, patient-centered communication in medical interactions is well established in the literature, but routine enactment of this approach is not universal among providers or patients in clinical settings.

The relationship between physicians and patients plays a crucial role in patients' health outcomes (Street et al., 2003). Medical encounters have been characterized by control, role negotiation, health-care commitment, trust, and time and money issues (Walker et al., 2001). Overall, communication research in medical visits has concluded that about 66 percent of talk in these interactions is biomedically focused (Roter et al., 1997). Patients who desire two-way communication in health-care interactions still may not be willing to assume control, and some research indicates physicians are as much as six times more willing than patients to assume control of the encounter (von Friederichs-Fitzwater and Gilgun, 2001). Physicians are typically able to achieve relational control of the medical encounter by focusing on the disease, changing topics, asking more questions, and talking more than the patient (von Friederichs-Fitzwater and Gilgun, 2001).

As discussed in chapter 3, on "patient characteristics," today patients often prefer a more patient-centered approach (Epstein and Street, 2007). A positive and communicative physician–patient relationship is imperative since this will lead to more patient involvement in the decision-making process (Beck, Daughtridge, and Sloan, 2002).

Doctors have significant influence on patient involvement based on the types of messages they employ, but this does not mean that patient involvement depends completely on the doctor (Street et al., 2005). Providers must identify different strategies to adapt to a patient's participation style, but this process requires sensitivity to learn about the patient's information needs, and flexibility to adapt communication based on those needs (Brown et al., 2002). Unique knowledge of the patient's desire for information allows providers to treat each patient as an individual, rather than one of many patients seen in a given day (Eldh, Ekman, and Enfohrs, 2006). Providers then adapt their messages to meet the needs of the patient. One example is the way in which providers inform patients of a cancer diagnosis. For some patients, a phone call explaining the news is helpful to give the patient time to seek familial support and compile questions to ask the provider during the follow-up consultation. However, other patients will prefer to receive a cancer diagnosis in the privacy of their provider's office (Lewis, 2009).

Sometimes providers use decision-making tools to engage patients and help explain scientific information about important medical issues (Street, 2007). Tools such as these can legitimate patient participation and help the provider focus the structure of a medical interview (Street, 2007). Patients may feel an enhanced sense of self-efficacy and an increased understanding of the risks and benefits of such issues as whether to use contraceptives at all, or which type of contraceptive might be most beneficial for a particular person or situation. For instance, a survey in Quebec in 2007 revealed that almost all physicians believe that having patients participate in developing their treatment plans and monitoring their state of health is a winning approach that will result in a better health care; 95 percent of the physicians believe that patients are better informed and 96 percent state that, as part of their practice, they talk to their patients about ways to improve their knowledge.

Providers' message content

The verbal content of medical encounters is comprised of several categories of messages from providers, including information giving and seeking, partnership-building, and supportive talk (Roter and Hall, 1993; Street et al., 2005). *Information giving* includes offering instruction, opinion, general information, and explanation about such topics as self-care, the nature and type of illness, diet, exercise, lifestyle choices, and answers to other questions (Roter and Hall, 1993; Street, et al., 2005). Doctors are often expected to extract key pieces of information from mountains of research on a given medical condition and convey that information to the patient in an easily digestible sound byte. Patients typically trust their provider to give accurate information, so the amount and type of information providers are expected to command is vast (Rutten and Arora, 2007). Utterances are in declarative form, and are intended to give medical and related information (e.g., "You need to increase your exercise level up to 30 minutes a day and it is time to engage in portion control with each meal. Aim for 4–5 small meals a day with a handful of protein and lots of leafy greens and colorful vegetables. Take Prilosec daily for the next 30 days and come back to see me in 6 weeks.").

Information seeking occurs when providers ask for specific information about patients' behaviors, adherence to treatment, concerns, or medical history. Utterances are either in the form of open- or closed-ended questions, and can be broad (e.g., "What do you know about pancreatic cancer?") or narrow ("How many times have you skipped taking your medication in the last month?") attempts to learn more about the patient (Roter and Hall, 1993; Street, et al., 2005).

Partnership-building includes messages that solicit, encourage, or affirm patients' efforts to express their opinions, ask questions, talk about their feelings, and participate in decision-making (Roter and Hall, 1993; Street et al., 2005). Providers may reflect on patients' narratives, or seek patients' opinions (e.g., "What do you think about that?" "Is this treatment something that appeals to you?" "Do you want to try this for now and we can reassess in a few months to see if you want to go ahead with surgery?" "Tell me more about your thoughts on that.").

Supportive talk includes verbal behaviors that agree, show approval, validate or support the patient's emotional or motivational state (Roter and Hall, 1993; Street et al., 2005). Supportive talk can include expressions of empathy for the patient, but in general it is any communication that encourages or supports the patient's situation or feelings (e.g., "That must be very hard on you and your family." "Congratulations on losing weight!" "Don't worry. It will be OK." "You are doing a fabulous job. Keep up the progress!"). Other less frequent types of verbal messages include negative talk and general social conversation. Negative talk (Roter and Hall, 1993) involves messages that express disagreement, disappointment, confrontation, or antagonism toward the patient. Social conversations are casual greetings and remarks often used to begin the conversation. Neither negative talk nor social conversation comprises much of the talk in medical encounters.

Gender differences

Research is inconclusive on the role of the gender of the patient in the type of language used in the medical encounter. Male doctors use similar language with male and female patients, but are more likely to ask female patients about their feelings or opinions than male patients. Nurse practitioners spend as much as two thirds of their patient interaction time engaged in interpersonal communication, and therefore have developed various patient-centered and partnership-building communication styles; however, almost 70 percent use a provider-centered communication style (Berry, 2009). Female patients may also be more conversational with their providers, and may therefore get more psychosocial information from their providers in return (Koehn et al., 2007).

Provider listening

CASE: In December 1999, a three-month-old Michigan infant died from acute hepatitis B. The infant's mother was chronically infected with hepatitis B and tested positive for hepatitis B surface antigen during her pregnancy. Unfortunately, the test results were communicated inaccurately to the hospital where the baby was born because the hospital pediatrician who was caring for the baby was not actively listening to the conversation when he wrote a note in the chart that indicated the infant's mother was "negative for hepatitis." As a result, the infant received no hepatitis B vaccine and no hepatitis B immune globulin (HBIG). To further complicate matters, neither the prenatal care provider nor the laboratory that did the prenatal testing communicated the positive result to the local health department as required by Michigan law. The infant became ill at about age three months and died less than two weeks after the onset of symptoms.

Adapted from case: Michigan Department of Community Health, "Three-month-old baby dies of acute hepatitis B," *Michigan Immunization Update* 7/2 (2000):1–2

When a physician or other provider is a poor communicator, medical mistakes are more likely to occur. In fact, medical mistakes are the eighth most common cause of deaths in the United States (McNeill and Walton, 2002). The US Institute of Medicine statistics report that as many as 98,000 patients die from preventable causes in the US each year (Kohn, Corrigan, and Donaldson, 2000). Preventable deaths are more common than the combined total of annual deaths from suicide, car accidents, airplane crashes, drowning, and poisoning (Barach and Small, 2000).

Although doctors are often expected to be infallible, medical mistakes do occur (Petronio, 2006). There are multiple causes of medical mistakes, such as fatigue, lack of training, stress, and distraction, but many errors occur from providers' ineffective communication (Firth-Cozens, 1993), including poor listening skills. Research suggests that when a patient is stressed or emotional (e.g., if bereaved of a loved one), helpful provider listening behaviors may be to just be present, both physically and emotionally, and to let the patient tell their story and share their feelings in the process (Lehman, Ellard and Wortman, 1986). Supportive listening by providers is most often accompanied by direct eye contact, and gives an appearance of actively accepting and processing what the patient says (Miller, Berg, and Archer, 1983).

Mistakes that could be alleviated through improved communication occur from unsuccessful interactions between patients and providers, and among health-care team members. Medical mistakes are often the result of a sequence of communicative errors. Errors may occur when a physician is in unfamiliar circumstances, uninformed, or when a doctor fails to engage in active listening. In turn, poor listening may trigger an incorrect treatment plan due to knowledge-based errors or skill-based errors (Ferner and Aronson, 2000). Knowledge-based errors are mistakes that occur when the provider does not have the complete knowledge to make correct decisions, such as when a provider chooses the wrong medication because s/he did not listen fully to the patient's symptoms. Skill-based errors occur when doctors have lapses of memory or make simple mistakes, such as those that might occur as a result of a lack of active engagement in the care process (Ferner and Aronson, 2000).

It is crucial that providers feel comfortable talking to one another about their opinions and hunches regarding any given medical case. Sometimes the medical hierarchy gets in the way of sound medical decision-making. For example, in Austria, the Professional Association of Gynecologists organized a seminar about communication, conducted by pilots. They presume that, every year, between 3,000 and 5,000 patients die in Austrian hospitals because of dysfunctional communication, inefficient teamwork, and cultural misunderstanding. Professor Pateiski, member of the board of the association and professor at the University of Vienna, suggests that physicians and members of the provider team use checklists as pilots do and eliminate the typically hierarchical way of communicating in a clinical environment (<http://www.informationhospitaliere. com/actualite-4990-medecins-prennent-cours-communication-pilotes-ligne.html>).

Even when communication does occur, all too often it is focused on the verbal content of the interaction as opposed to a full exploration of both verbal and non-verbal content. Seminal research in the importance of non-verbal communication in the way a receiver interprets a message reveals spoken words only account for 30–35 percent of the perceived meaning. The rest is transmitted through non-verbal communication that can only be detected through visual and auditory listening (Birdwhistell, 1970). Positive non-verbal behaviors from providers may include gazes and head nods (Beck et al., 2002). In most conversations, 55 percent of the meaning is translated non-verbally, while at least 38 percent is indicated by the tone of voice, and only 7 percent is conveyed by the words used (Mehrabian, 1981). All too often, providers are filling out forms or reading notes from previous encounters, and therefore they completely miss important non-verbal and paralinguistic cues from the patient.

A pediatrician recounted the story of an intelligent, caring mother who brought her young son in to the office for an unknown illness (Bronfin, 2008). The doctor could not seem to find anything wrong with the child as he went through the regular mental checklist of the examination. This particular doctor was especially attuned to the subtlety of communication, however, so he sensed something was wrong based on the mother's persistent non-verbal communication. Finally, the mother pulled the doctor aside and asked if it was harmful to her son to see his father hit her (Bronfin, 2008).

This example highlights the importance of listening and observing the verbal and non-verbal cues from patients and their families. There is comfort in having and using a checklist or script of "steps" for the medical interview, but providers who actively listen to their patients are more likely to pick up on important information that will be missed if the provider is not actively engaged in the verbal and non-verbal content of the interaction.

Both providers and patients can use the following three simple solutions to connecting verbally and non-verbally during medical interactions:

1   *Focus.* It can be hard sometimes to get past the setting and the circum-
    stances of a doctor visit, but focusing on the goals of the visit can help
    make it more successful. Patients and providers should try to give
    complete attention to the person speaking and the information or
    question being conveyed. Most people think faster than speakers can
    talk, which is one of the reasons why our minds can often wander when
    we are trying to listen. Focusing on the other person means actively
    listening, not thinking about what to say next.

2   *Feedback.* Effective feedback to patients includes expressions of empa-
    thy and supportive communication. Providing feedback is extremely
    beneficial, and feedback can be delivered as either verbal or non-verbal
    cues. Sometimes important medical information is missed because
    doctors are so busy they forget to let patients speak. Patients who wish
    to politely interject can wait until there is a break in their speaking
    rhythm, then use verbal and non-verbal communication to actively
    engage the provider. Both patients and providers can add clarity to
    their interactions by summarizing key points, asking clarifying ques-
    tions, and speaking words of encouragement. Although excessive verbal
    communication can add to the length of an appointment, providers
    who engage in active listening may actually save time by correctly
    assessing the patient's needs. The pediatrician in the story mentioned
    earlier could have wasted more time trying to find something wrong
    with the child, but he was tuned in to the non-verbal cues of the mother
    so he was able to get to the point of the visit. Being fully present in any
    interaction can help both parties use feedback to quickly move to the
    most important information.

3   *Filtering.* Despite the fact that many health-care providers choose
    their profession because they care deeply about helping others, the
    dehumanization of patients is a common part of medical educa-
    tion (Bronfin, 2008). Typical examples of dehumanizing stereotyping
    patients include reaching conclusions about a patient's current medi-
    cal needs based on staff comments, previous encounters, or cultural
    stereotypes (Bronfin, 2008). Although doctors and patients do not
    always look alike, sound alike, or have the same goals for a health-care
    interaction, it is important to filter out judgments about the speaker or
    what s/he is saying. Putting aside preconceived biases and listening
    to everything being said aids in creating a collaborative and honest
    relationship.

Provider emotion

While modern medicine is aided by a dazzling array of technologies, like
high-resolution MRI scans and pinpoint DNA analysis, language is still
the bedrock of clinical practice. Typically, it is the doctor who assesses
our emotional state. But few of us realize how strongly a physician's mood
and temperament influence his medical judgment. We, of course, may
get only glimpses of our doctor's feelings, but even those brief moments

can reveal a great deal about why he chose to pursue a possible diagnosis or offered a particular treatment.

Groopman, 2007: 8

Empathy reassures patients that they are being taken care of and this understanding helps them process the information given by the provider (Ulene, 2009).

The science of medicine is taught in medical schools, but learning to be a physician is not only about new knowledge and skills; it is also a process of learning what it means to be a medical professional (Wagner et al., 2007). Sometimes medical students who are competent communicators in their own lives need specific training on how to translate interpersonal skills they may already possess to the medical encounter. For example, imagine the frightening feeling of being a parent of a baby who has suddenly become extremely ill. When taking the baby to hospital, it is difficult to be calm or think rationally. It becomes the responsibility of a good health-care team to care for the child, but to do so they need the parent's cooperation.

Medical residents greatly benefit from receiving actual training on how to handle such situations, and those who receive interpersonal skills training are more likely to successfully adapt their communication when working with parents in a pediatric setting (Hart et al., 2006). Specific messages that are most effective when interacting with concerned parents of a sick child are those that include an increase in the use of praise, empathy, and collaboration with families (Hart et al., 2006). Patients feel it is essential for health-care providers to possess the ability to communicate in an informative, humane, and accurate manner (Wensinga et al., 1999), and therefore these skills could be emphasized in medical school curriculums. Despite the lack of emphasis on verbal, non-verbal, and listening skills training in medical schools, there is significant evidence that such training can increase providers' use of messages offering praise, empathy, and collaboration with patients and caregivers. Moreover, even a brief course in communication skills training can increase patient satisfaction and improve overall perceptions of care (Hart et al., 2006).

When discussing the lack of training of medical students on the topic of dealing with emotion, physician Loren Stephen explained:

> If the emotional dilemmas encountered by medical students in training are disregarded or dealt with only incidentally or accidentally, the students will stumble in their desperation into the maladaptive roles seen all around us in graduate physicians. The students will meet these issues by transmuting their patients into abstractions, which offer neither the pain nor gratification of human intimacy. They will take refuge from human responsibility in obsessive attention to detail. (Korsch and Harding, 1997: 145)

Traditionally, medical schools seek to socialize students into a profession that emphasizes withholding emotional responses to patients' pain and suffering (Korsch and Harding, 1997). From the time that students begin working with cadavers, they are trained to disassociate themselves from feelings about the process of medicine. For example, dissecting a formerly living human sometimes necessitates the use of dark humor to cope with the traumatic experience of cutting and examining a dead body. Dehumanization continues as medical interns endure grueling work schedules, morbidity, mortality, and difficult interactions with patients, caregivers, and co-workers. A culture of dehumanization can exist within hospital and medical training facilities, so medical residents and interns often learn to communicate based on that approach to medical care (Korsch and Harding, 1997).

Because of the lack of focus on the importance of interpersonal communication training in medical schools, there have been calls to include tests of traits like empathy when screening medical school applicants (Hemmerdinger, Stoddart, and Lilford, 2007). Measuring potential medical students' abilities to exhibit empathy with patients might be a good way to predict how they will interact with patients and family members, such as distraught parents of a sick baby. These tests could also be the first step to creating more comprehensive communication training, including empathy, for medical residents and other health-care professionals.

This perspective puts doctors' abilities to connect with patients on par with academic records and standardized test scores when selecting potential medical students. Should medical students be tested and assessed based on their communication skills? Similarly, does it seem a good idea for SATs and high school GPAs to be supplemented with an interpersonal communication skills test for admission into all colleges? Would such a test be a helpful indicator of potential success? How are these two situations similar or different?

Breaking bad news

Perhaps the most emotionally difficult communication that providers must master is breaking bad news in an empathetic and comforting manner (Rob, 2009; Sparks et al., 2007). Patients create opportunities for providers to express empathy during medical interactions, even when they are relatively unfamiliar with the physician, but physicians most often deal with the opportunity by acknowledging the situation without really sharing their own experiences or feelings (Bylund and MaKoul, 2005). Direct communication of the basic bad news message focuses on the topic itself, as opposed to the social or emotional implications of the message for the patient or provider (Sparks et al., 2007). Empathic communication can bolster patients' views of a provider's communication competence, and usually expresses understanding for the patient's feelings, without actually sharing the patient's emotions (Hemmerdinger, Stoddard, and Lilford, 2007). Beach et al. (2004) found that physicians rarely self-disclose at all in medical encounters, and disclosure of personal feelings is rare. Providers tend to use a direct style of delivering bad news.

Despite this, Wanzer, Booth-Butterfield, and Gruber (2004) found that non-verbal immediacy, listening, clarity, and empathic communication were important predictors of patient satisfaction. There are strong indications that patients' communication and relationship with their care providers can also profoundly reduce emotional distress when receiving news that must be grieved, when coping with a disease, and when reframing the concept of hope (Butow et al., 1996; Evans et al., 2006; Roter et al., 1995). Naming and acknowledging patient and family emotions early on in a diagnosis/prognosis, and utilizing communication techniques that are open-ended, are more likely to invite a patient to share anxieties. Put simply, the perspective of the other is recognized in the production of comfort messages (Zimmerman and Applegate, 1992). Addressing emotions also aligns physicians with their patients/families before challenging decisions are made together (Tulsky, 2005; Rabow, Hauser, and Adams, 2004).

Despite these findings, research on communication training protocols designed to assist medical students with the delivery of terminal bad news has revealed contradictory conceptualizations, and it has been argued that communicating a terminal prognosis requires adaptive communication based on the patient's acceptability (Wittenberg-Lyles et al., 2008).

SPIKES

One example of a commonly used set of steps (or script) for communicating with patients is the SPIKES model. SPIKES, an acronym for Setting, Perception, Invitation, Knowledge, Empathy, and Summary, is a protocol that is commonly used in the medical school curriculum to train students to deliver bad news, including terminal bad news. According to the SPIKES protocol, *setting* guides the physician to create the best physical circumstances for conferencing with the patient; the details of the protocol even address proxemics, non-verbal leakage, and the presence of family in the conference space. *Perception* addresses the "ask before you tell" principle; physicians are to assess patients' understanding of their own medical situations. *Invitation* asks patients how much information they would like to have concerning their diagnosis/prognosis. *Knowledge* is the step in which physicians actually impart "bad" news. Alignment with the patient is encouraged in this step, as well as the use of non-technical language in small units of meaning. *Empathy* follows the breaking of the bad news; here the physician is encouraged to listen for and identify the emotions of the patient and identify the cause of those emotions – making a connection between the two. The intention here is to validate the patient's feelings and experience. The final element in the protocol is to summarize and strategize a plan for the next step of care (Baile et al., 2000).

The SPIKES originator, Robert Buckman, asserts that SPIKES is not a script, but is a structured performance meant to take place in a particular context and order. Buckman has provided a path for physicians to follow, though the wording they select can take many forms. SPIKES is intended in the best interest of physicians, to relieve their stress related to delivering bad news. We experience stress when we are in difficult situations and when we have to process too much information at one time. When used in conjunction with simulated breaking bad news training scenarios, the SPIKES model has been shown to significantly improve medical students' appearances, communication strategies, and emotional control in these situations (Bowyer et al., 2009).

A communication-based tool for breaking bad news was adapted from SPIKES to more prominently reflect the reciprocal nature of creating shared meaning (Villagran, Weathers, Keefe, and Sparks, 2010). The COMFORT model extends SPIKES by using interaction adaptation theory (IAT) (Burgoon, Stern, and Dillman, 1995) to more fully explain the process of mutual influence between patient and provider (Duggan and Bradshaw, 2008), and to demonstrate how the evolution of communication events such as a BBN occur based on the perceptions of the power structure of the interaction. In IAT, the matching response, or *norm of reciprocity* (Gouldner, 1960), evolves as patients and clinicians adapt to each other based on the types of verbal and non-verbal messages received, and their own changing needs within the interaction (Duggan and Bradshaw, 2008).

COMFORT, which builds on existing protocols such as SPIKES, is an acronym for seven competencies to be taught/practiced through specific communication skills (Villagran, Weathers, Keefe, and Sparks, 2010). COMFORT serves as the framework for breaking bad news and stands for: *communication, orientation, mindfulness, family, ongoing, reiterative messages,* and *team.* COMFORT is not a linear guide for BBN performance by clinicians, but rather a set of competencies that should occur reflexively and concurrently by patients, family members, and providers. The COMFORT process is in line with basic communication principles because it allows for more mirroring, reciprocity, family/audience inclusion, and more adaptive dialogue based on the needs of the patient.

Improving patient understanding

Although SPIKES is designed for breaking bad news to patients, there are several other approaches to structuring patient interactions. Providers who seek to verify patient understanding of diagnosis or treatment information often employ the *Teach Back* method to engage patients in verbal interaction (Rowan, 2008). Teach Back is frequently used to help patients remember specific concepts or instructions. Patients listen to information, and then teach it back to their provider in their own words. This method allows providers to ensure a patient fully understands medical instructions.

Providers should not treat Teach Back as a test, but rather as an opportunity for clarification and shared understanding (Rowan, 2008). A provider might say, for example, "What will you tell your husband about our discussion?" or "I just gave you a lot of information. What do you view as the most important things we have discussed?" When a patient cannot recall or states incorrect information, the provider has another opportunity to make the information more memorable or clear. Providers who use Teach Back can also create an opportunity for additional questions from the patient.

A final structural approach to provider–patient interactions is called Ask Me Three (Partnership for Clear Health Communication, 2006). This approach encourages patients to ask three common questions in each medical encounter. Providers should always structure the medical encounter to ensure that by the end of their conversation the patient clearly understands the answers to the following:

1 What is my main problem?
2 What do I need to do?
3 Why is it important for me to do this?

As medicine becomes more complex, it is harder for an individual clinician to provide all the information that a specific patient may need or want, but these three questions provide a good framework for basic understanding.

Health message construction

We must begin to construct tailored health messages "where people are" in their own communities as well as within their interpersonal relationships and social networks; this may range from bedside to the physician's office, to places where family and friends gather, from the morning water cooler or coffee shop to the afternoon shopping spree, school, office, or set of appointments. As with recent calls for personalized approaches to medicine, health communication scholars are calling for an integration of interpersonal-based personalized messaging, stating that we should construct and tailor interpersonal and mediated messages in a systematic, understandable way for each patient and his or her unique characteristics (e.g., Sparks and Nussbaum, 2008).

Designing and delivering health communication messages to match the specific communication skills, needs, and predispositions of the targeted population is a crucial component of health-care delivery (Sparks and Nussbaum, 2008). The strategic use of health communication has been found to reduce health risks, incidence, morbidity, and mortality, while enhancing quality of life across the continuum of cancer care (prevention, detection, diagnosis, treatment, survivorship, and end-of-life care) (see, e.g., Byock, 2000; Hiatt and Rimer, 1999; Wenzel et al., 2005).

Conclusion

As trained experts in their field, health-care providers serve a unique and important role in society. They are the glue to the health-care interaction as they are the highly trained experts with extensive technical knowledge and experience. There is strong evidence that providers conducting medical interviews must be taught to recognize the problems and issues embedded in interview data that can be concealed by humorous communicative cues and anecdotes, patient self-disclosure, and storytelling. Situations where humor, self-disclosures, and/or narratives surface in the medical encounter are often subtle hints that can lead to better understanding of the problems at hand. Among other things, the interviewee may not be conscious of his or her effort to convey important information via, for example, humor. For some, the disguise of humor may also be serving as a protective shield in the communication exchange. Effective health and human service providers and researchers know how complex and challenging it can be to obtain complete and accurate information from individuals who have much information to share and many emotional barriers to overcome in a communication process.

Discussion Questions for Providers to Encourage Patient Participation

How health-care providers word questions can have a strong influence on the responses that patients provide. By using specific language, providers can empower patients and encourage open communication. Open-ended questions are especially useful for allowing the patient to define the conversation.

> How can I help you today?
> Can you tell me more about your shoulder pain (or whatever problem they mention)?
> I'm curious to know more about . . .
> That must have been (very painful/frustrating/emotional) . . .
> With your permission I would like to conduct some further tests (or whatever else needs to be done).
> What do you know already? What do you want to know more about?
> How does this treatment plan fit with what you've been thinking?

5 Caregiving Characteristics

My friend Vickie came into my office today for a meeting. We had a chance to catch up after the meeting and I asked Vickie about her current work/family situation.

"I'm working as a caregiver for my father-in-law these days," Vickie said. "He has late stage Parkinson's disease and requires help with everything. We have a lift to get him in and out of bed; I've got to care for his catheter; it's just a lot of work."

I asked her how many hours each week she spent helping her mother-in-law, assuming that she traveled to their home for a few hours each day.

"That's the hard part," she said. "They live with us. The caregiving never ends – I can't begin to count how many hours each week I work."

She was excited to be out of the house for the meeting as it was just about the only break she could see on the horizon.

As I listened to Vickie I heard what I hear so often from family caregivers: the work is not only physically challenging, but emotionally draining as well.

It's hard to be the "rock" that your family relies on. It's exhausting, no matter how much help you get from other members of the family.

Vickie's husband, mother-in-law, son, and grandchildren are all involved in Grandpa's care. But at the end of the day, the person they all turn to is the one with the experience and training as a caregiver – Vickie. And of course, Vickie being the person that she is, worries about them all even when she's not there.

Posted by Sharon K. Brothers, April 8, 2009; available at: <http://caringformomanddad.blogspot.com/2009/04/caregiving-takes-emotional-toll-on.html>

This chapter explores various communication issues related to caregiving, including communication needs of caregivers and recipients, family decision-making, and aspects of palliative care and hospice care. It also touches on some of the most delicate issues involved with end-of-life decision-making, death, and dying. The chapter pays special attention to the unique emerging aspects of distance caregiving, which will probably increase as our society becomes more and more mobile. Caregiving is a crucial component of patient and provider interaction because health care usually involves the loved ones in addition to the patient. Caregivers often serve in mediator roles between formal providers and patients. Caregivers typically take on an informal provider role too, as they learn the ropes about caring for their loved ones, often helping them to navigate and dissect the mounds of health information and subsequent decision-making that stems from patient and provider interaction.

Caregiving is one of the most difficult yet rewarding processes one may experience and will likely impact each individual, or a family member or friend, at some point across everyone's life span. As with becoming a parent for the first time, most of us are not prepared for the relatively unknown challenges that are likely to emerge when entering this unknown territory of caregiving. A caregiver is defined as an adult who currently or recently (i.e., in the past 12 months) has assisted someone over the age of 50 with at least one Activity of Daily Living (ADL) such as giving medications and getting dressed, and two or more Instrumental Activities of Daily Living (IADLs), including housework, arranging and supervising services, and managing finances (Koerin and Harrigan, 2002). Governmental and societal structures tend to encourage informal caregiving of their aging populations (Clarke, 1995; Finch and Mason, 1993). In 1995, family caregiving saved Britain approximately £40 billion (Baillie, 2007). Despite this governmental and societal encouragement, family caregiving is unpaid, can continue for a lengthy time period, is an almost constant time commitment (Baillie, 2007), and is a passive decision if the caregiver believes there is no one else or no other alternative (Brereton and Nolan, 2000).

Adult children are generally considered to be the most important and frequent providers of informal care to their older adult parents (Connidis and Kemp, 2008; Hogan, Eggebeen, and Clogg, 1993; NAC/MMMI, 2004; Smith, 1998; Stafford, 2005) and an older adult's interactions about health care are often intergenerational in nature (Nussbaum and Fisher, 2009).

A 2009 study by an American Association of Retired Persons (AARP) of caregiving in the United States conducted telephone interviews with 1,480 caregivers aged 18 and older, including samples of approximately 200 African-Americans, 200 Hispanics, and 200 Asian Americans. The extensive study found that caregivers of younger adults, older adults, and children with special needs consist of 29 percent of the US adult population, that is, 65.7 million people identify themselves as caregivers, which includes 31 percent of all households, on average providing 20 hours of care per week (see <www.aarp.org>). Further, among caregivers aged 18 and older, the average caregiver's age is 49 and the average age of the care recipient is 69, with the modern-day caregiver still likely to be mainly female (66 percent).

Caregiving, including being a caregiver of children, lasts an average of 4.6 years (AARP, 2009). AARP also reports an increase in the proportion of caregivers who need more help and information regarding caregiving issues. Despite most caregivers reporting they experience minor physical strain, emotional stress, or financial hardship as a result of being a caregiver, there are signs that caregiving is becoming more emotionally stressful for some and that many are experiencing more financial hardship in fulfilling the difficult and complex caregiving role than five years ago (AARP). Communication plays a key role in the caregiving experience in terms of instrumental and emotional support. Clearly, more evidence-based research is needed in this important area as our population ages and government becomes less reliable for families, which will indeed force families to take on stronger roles in caring for each other emotionally, financially, physically, and instrumentally in terms of daily needs. Family caregivers are important sources of information about patient behaviors, and they are often crucial in terms of communicating information about pain to providers (Pecchioni and Sparks, 2007). Caregivers are usually family members and friends who do not get paid for the care provided. The majority of dependent older adults in the United States who require long-term assistance currently receive care from family members (Sparks-Bethea, 2002). The number of lay caregivers is likely to increase within the next few decades due to a number of factors, including, but not limited to, increases in average life span, as well as advances in medical technologies extending the lives of those individuals with long-term illnesses (Sparks, Travis, and Thompson, 2005; Travis and Sparks-Bethea, 2001; Travis, Sparks-Bethea, and Winn, 2000; Wright, Sparks, and O'Hair, 2008).

In order to achieve the most successful and effective caregiving experience for all involved, from disease detection, recovery, or end-of-life, effective communication is key. Research indicates that lay caregivers are often unprepared to deal with the many challenges of caregiving, and they can find it difficult to cope with the demands of providing care for family members and other loved ones (Andrews, 2001; Sarna and McCorkle, 1996). Many people feel uncomfortable talking about the various issues surrounding the daily activities of caregiving, and especially issues of death and dying. Because of this, and due to the high levels of emotion involved, many are not prepared to handle the issues that arise.

Caregiving and stress

How individuals accomplish the communicative act of caregiving can be quite stressful to all involved. Adult children and their aging parents are now more likely than ever before to move away from their families (Davidhizar, 1999; De Wit, Wister, and Burch, 1988; Finch and Mason, 1993), putting strain on family decision-making. People are living longer and the females in the family are increasingly joining the workforce, which leaves fewer family members available for daily care needs (Baillie, 2007). Perhaps most importantly, caregiving experiences are often transitional times for families who must adjust to new ways of interacting with each other, with new ways of behaving and decision-making, as they adjust in ways that enable them to manage stressful family changes and emerge resilient while remaining emotionally intact as a family.

Caregiving competence and social support

Caregivers often lack the wide array of communication skills needed to successfully meet the needs of the patient, as well as their own needs (Andrews, 2001; Bakas, et al., 2002; Wright, Sparks, and O'Hair, 2008). The ability to communicate competently is particularly crucial in the family caregiving context, as research indicates a link among family communication, health, and adjustment to diseases such as cancer (Helgeson and Cohen, 1999; Sparks, 2008). Communication competence refers to the ability to construct and use effective messages to meet one's needs and goals and to successfully create and maintain satisfying relationships (Wiemann, 1977). Research indicates that caregivers with higher communication competence had lower perceived stress levels and higher satisfaction with their support networks (Query and Wright, 2003).

Formal health-care providers typically handle medical patient needs, whereas informal caregivers (usually a family member) take on a number of tasks, including providing emotional support, transportation, managing finances, monitoring symptoms, coordinating schedules, increased housework, and running errands, and this so-called caregiver burden takes a toll on caregivers in the long run (Andrews, 2001; Laizner et al., 1993). These activities can lead to physical and emotional exhaustion for the caregiver who sees a constant decline in the health of their loved one. In fact, 17 percent of caregivers consider their health to be fair or poor, compared to 13 percent of the general adult population (AARP, 2009).

Caregivers' communication with their social network and providers can have a positive impact on their stress levels, particularly when they are able to use their communication skills to obtain assistance and emotional support (Wright, Sparks, and O'Hair, 2008). Current research suggests that caregivers who are able to express their feelings about the caregiving situation report better quality of life than those who do not have these opportunities (Tamayo et al., 2010). In addition, many caregivers have found the use of humor to be an effective way of coping with the complexities of caregiving, as it often provides relief from the stresses involved in the caregiving process (Harzold and Sparks, 2007; Sparks, Travis, and Thompson, 2005; Sparks-Bethea, Travis, and Pecchioni, 2000).

Caregiving and communicative cues

Professionals who depend on interview situations to gather information about long and often complex family histories may be surprised at how often the interactants use humor to help them through difficult conversations. When interviewees receive favorable reactions about their humorous stories, it increases their confidence and motivation to reveal important and usually more sensitive information about their health-care experiences (Sparks et al., 2005). In all cases, it is assumed that the interviewer has first established a relational connection with the interviewee on some level. The responsibility for gathering information that lies just past the humor cue rests with the interviewer. It is his or her responsibility to pay close attention to the placement and timing of the cues and to develop the probes that will keep the caregiver from moving too quickly past the object of the humorous account.

What follows is a hypothetical exchange from Sparks, Travis and Thompson (2005) that is based on actual conversations with informal providers, who are often long-term family caregivers. In this exchange, the caregiver is a 72-year-old wife of a gentleman with moderate dementia who has recently become sexually aggressive around their female friends. The wife asked her case manager to come to the house so she could discuss his care arrangements and the long-term care options that might be available to her in the future. During this telephone conversation, she vaguely mentioned that he has been having some non-specific behavioral changes that she believes are related to his progressive dementia.

The wife begins the interview with general information about his condition and what their typical day is like. A comfortable level of conversation is established. When asked if she is having any specific problems she replies:

> "Well, you know how men are. He sees a pretty woman and he is just all over her" (*smiling at the interviewer and laughs softly*). "He has always been such a lady's man!" (*big chuckle*) "His latest move is trying to kiss our female friends on the lips when he sees them. You can just imagine how much they like that old man coming after them!" (*smiles and chuckles*)

In this case, the caregiver may not even be aware that he or she is using humor in the conversation. An appropriate response for the case manager in our scenario is:

> "Let's talk about your husband's attraction to your female friends. Can you give me some other examples of how he behaves around them?"

This method of communication is very likely to be a face-saving effort on the part of the wife before she shares more troubling or embarrassing information about her husband's sexual overtures (Sparks, Travis and Thompson, 2005). The development of probing questions that do not upset the caregiver and give the interviewer factual information is both an art and a science. The skilled interviewer in this situation may smile during these comments, but he or she knows that the humor in the message is both a defense mechanism and a convenient, non-threatening communication vehicle.

One common pitfall that novice providers and interviewers encounter is to try and make the caregiver feel more comfortable by swapping similar "funny stories" that others have shared. Although these types of exchanges keep both interviewer and interviewee at a reasonable level of social comfort, because they are both avoiding the real issue – sexual aggression – they are not effective communication processes. At some point, the caregiver must be given an opportunity to disclose the serious or troubling information that she needs to share. Our case manager is practicing appropriate communication responses with the following response.

> "Although I see you smiling when you describe your husband's behavior, I wonder if it isn't also causing you some discomfort and distress around your friends."

Finding the message that is really being delivered and doing what needs to be done to understand that message in the context of the caregiver's story have to be the responsibility of the professional interviewer (Sparks et al., 2005).

Family decision-making

The family is a complex unit comprised of individuals with varied cognitive, emotional, and behavioral characteristics and abilities that can greatly affect family decision-making across an individual's life span (Sparks, 2008). "Decision-making" describes the process by which families make choices, judgments, and ultimately come to conclusions that guide behaviors (Sparks, 2008). Family decision-making implies that more than one member's input and agreement is involved (Scanzoni and Polonko, 1980). In the decision-making process, families can acknowledge the differences among members and negotiate their needs for closeness and independence (Baxter and Montgomery, 1996).

Family decisions are negotiated every day from family decisions in the childhood and adolescent years to middle- and later-life family decisions, many of which occur in health-care environments. Family decision processes in the health-care environment are particularly difficult and complex because of the uncertainties, emotions, technical language, and subsequent health outcomes (e.g., Sparks, 2003b). Conflicting information from various sources can be difficult to navigate and process to make the most informed health-care decisions. Families make decisions about health issues using information from a variety of sources, including insurance provider lists, Internet research, recommendations from primary care physicians and specialists, interpersonal communication with friends and family members, and mediated messages (see Pecchioni and Sparks, 2007).

Family decision-making has become increasingly complex as family life has dramatically changed over the last several decades. Changing roles of women, increasing integration of women in the labor force, increases in divorce rates, increased mobility, increased longevity, and complex health-care environments are just some of the crucial changes that are impacting families and thus, arguably, impacting family decision-making across the life span (Sparks, 2008). The intricacies of the caregiving context increase these complexities dramatically for contemporary families. Significant research has indicated that serious illness impacts the lives of ill individuals, their families, and loved ones (Ballard-Reisch, 1996; McCubbin and McCubbin, 1991; Rait and Lederberg, 1989; Sparks, 2008), to the extent that some have argued that serious illness is a "family issue" (Hardwig, 1990; Sparks, 2007, 2008).

Not surprisingly, differing family structures often impact management of the illness (Sparks, 2008). Dynamics in dual-parent families, single-parent families, and blended families vary. For example, Anderson (1998) found differences in communication patterns and predictors of family dysfunction for dual-parent and single-parent families. Family structures also differ by culture and immigrant assimilation. Recent research suggests that Latinos value a more collaborative, family-centered approach to caregiving decision-making, and those who have immigrated more recently, as compared to those who immigrated longer ago, are more likely to make care decisions that are consistent with family values without consulting the care recipient first (Radina, Gibbons, and Lim, 2009).

One area of caregiving research that health communication scholars have focused upon is decision-making conversations between adult children and their older adult parents, which are typically not explicit, collaborative, or planned prior to parent dependency (Fowler and Fisher, 2007; Pecchioni and Nussbaum, 2000). Specifically, Fowler and Fisher (2007) and Pecchioni and Nussbaum (2000) have linked these decision-making conversations to the concepts of autonomy, which involves having control over and responsibility for one's own life, and paternalism, which involves believing that an individual might impose a decision on someone else for that person's welfare. In prompted mother–daughter caregiving discussions prior to dependency, paternalistic daughters took control of the conversation (Pecchioni and Nussbaum, 2000). Further, for adult children, their beliefs in paternalism and shared autonomy positively predicted, and their independent autonomy negatively predicted, both their awareness of future parental care needs and the requirement for caregiving information (Fowler and Fisher, 2007). For aging parents, their beliefs in paternalism and shared autonomy predicted awareness of their future care needs (ibid.). Autonomy and paternalism are consistent informative variables in the understanding of the complex caregiving communication environment.

As the number of options for health-care delivery and treatment increases, decision-making about health-care issues has become more complex. Decades ago, a patient might visit one provider, who would communicate information about diagnosis and treatment protocols. Patients and families typically followed the instructions of one physician without sharing in most decisions, and without consultation with others. The twenty-first-century family often decides about health issues using information from a variety of sources, including insurance provider lists, Internet research, recommendations from primary care physicians and specialists, and interpersonal communication with friends and family members, as well as being greatly influenced by exposure to mediated messages (Sparks, 2008). Conflicting information from various sources can be difficult to navigate. Multiple sources of information can aid in making effective decisions, but the path to a clear health-care plan for families is complex. More information about a health concern often results in more options available, and, thus, the more decisions a patient may be faced with in the care process. Sound decision-making in health care relies on effective communication among providers, families, and other external sources of information, combined with the ability to process that information.

Message processing in the caregiving context

In order to implement more sound communicative practices during health care, it is crucial to understand that diagnoses are as complex as the patients being diagnosed. Every patient processes the uncertainties of health care in a unique manner. For example, developing the most effective communication to encourage detection and prevention of an impending health problem assumes that the patient will engage in message-relevant thinking (see, e.g., Sparks and Turner, 2008). That is, we create health messages hoping that the message will gain the attention of the audience, that the audience will actually read or listen to the message, and will then engage in thoughtful message processing. Early research on thoughtful processing of persuasive messages focused on issues such as the time and attention allocated to the message, the comprehension of the message content, and the acceptance of the message conclusions (Hovland, Janis, and Kelley, 1953; Todorov, Chaiken, and Henderson, 2002). Yet we know from research that although people can carefully process health messages, they do not always do so (Sparks, 2007, 2008; Sparks and Turner, 2008).

Individuals who process health messages systematically will think carefully about the message and engage in cognitive processing (or thinking) that is relevant to the message content. Human beings typically will invest only the necessary cognitive effort to complete the task at hand. In order to engage in systematic processing people must be sufficiently motivated, and have sufficient cognitive resources. Motivation is affected by how personally relevant the message is, as well as message exposure (Chaiken, 1980; Sparks and Turner, 2008).

Attitude change about risky or unhealthy behaviors that occurs due to systematic processing is much stronger, lasts longer, and has a better chance of future behavior change (Sparks, 2008; Sparks and Turner, 2008). If the arguments are perceived to be high quality, the message receiver should generate positive thoughts and there is a higher chance of persuasion. But if the message argument is perceived to be low quality, the thoughts generated by the message will be negative, leading to less persuasion. It is believed that if we can motivate careful processing, message receivers will engage in message elaboration and convince themselves to engage in the recommended actions so they will be more likely to engage in long-term change (Sparks, 2008). For caregivers, this may mean the difference between early detection of infection or additional illnesses with improved survival chances, or of failing to detect infections or illness with a greater likelihood of the patient dying.

As Sparks (2008) points out, these findings have tremendous implications for family health-care decision-making. For example, when a patient receives prognosis and treatment information from a provider, it is imperative that the message is cognitively processed by the patient and caregivers who are likely to be active participants in the decision-making processes. If the care recipient is motivated to make positive changes in unhealthy behaviors, he or she will be more likely to systematically process the information before making relevant decisions about potential behavior change.

Caregivers who feel uncertain about health issues will seek out additional information to assist them in making sound decisions. Generally, the decision-making process about what to do at the end of a patient's life requires members of the health-care team to meet and discuss options with the patient and the family. The role of the family in the decision-making process in these initial stages is particularly important, as the caregiving team is often comprised of the patient's family and loved ones (Connor et al., 2002).

Individual differences in message processing and the history of family member dynamics result in complex decision-making for caregivers. For terminally ill patients and family members probabilistic judgments might be the extent to which they accept a negative prognosis. Evaluative judgments might include individual perceptions of the patient's life or the relationships among family members. These two components are integrated in the minds of patients and family members through messages that are sent and received as part of the health-care experience (Babrow, 1992, 2001). Individual differences in decision-making strategies also have the potential to influence mental health. Anderson et al. (2009) found that relatives of ICU patients who chose to engage in passive decision-making about end-of-life care were more likely to have anxiety and be depressed than those who used more active strategies.

In a review of variables affecting family decision-making and family dynamics in later life, Rothchild (1994) found that a range of factors confront families as they decide about terminal care of a family member. Many families react to their sense of guilt and hopelessness by pushing for maximal medical intervention until the bitter end. This often results in patient failure to resist such pressure and persuasion, consequently accepting treatments that they very likely would not have chosen if left to themselves. Rothchild includes the following variables:

1   patient's role in the family (boss, scapegoat, caregiver);
2   ages of patient and family members;
3   family continuity and cohesion;
4   who is considered to be "family";
5   how information and decisions are shared within the family;
6   presence of denial, guilt, and anger;
7   communication of treatment wishes to proxies;
8   comfort with sophisticated technology;
9   ethnicity and religion; and
10   economic pressures.

Steps in talking with families about treatment withdrawal include:

1   keeping explanations simple until it is clear that more detail will be helpful rather than overwhelming;
2   asking them to summarize their understanding of what has been said;
3   recommending a plan rather than asking family to decide.

Conflict is most often addressed by:

1   convening a family meeting;
2   giving a simple, consistent description of the patient's condition and prognosis;

3   outlining in simple terms the specific areas for decision-making;
4   allowing the family time to discuss the issues, ask questions, and express an opinion;
5   nominating one family member to communicate with the treatment team; and
6   setting a deadline for the family to make a decision.

In sum, two scenarios frequently emerge: (1) the family pressures the patient to make specific care decisions (for example, the patient is pressurized by the family to keep fighting despite their wish to end treatments); or (2) family members disagree about health-care choices and the patient's decision impacts their own health care as well as their family system. All of these decisions are often frightening and difficult for families to sort through and to ultimately reach the best decision for the patient and family.

Family decisions are negotiated every day, from early family decisions in the adolescent years to later-life family decisions which often occur in health-care environments. As each patient and family member processes messages differently, decision-making can be a complex communicative process. Arguably, this is especially salient in end-of-life care as the patient and family are considered the unit of care. Overall, the role of the family is especially important in understanding how a patient makes health-care choices that most certainly impact the entire family.

Communication among family members may exhibit a number of changes when they take on caregiver roles (Sparks-Bethea, 2002; Williams and Nussbaum, 2001). Marital satisfaction can be damaged by the financial cost of providing for children and parents, as well as the emotional costs associated with the caregiving relationship. Married couples caring for a parent who report lower marital satisfaction report that the presence of a parent in the home reduces the amount of overall communication time within the marital dyad and the amount of private time between couples, as well as increasing certain types of communication between the couple, such as decision-making. These changes in communication appear to affect even long-term marriages, since they have been found to experience declines in marital satisfaction when the partners are caring for an aging parent (Sparks-Bethea, 2002).

Distance caregiving

Recent research by Bevan and Sparks (2010) looks at the relatively unknown communicative context of distance caregiving by considering long-distance caregiving (LDC) as a context that combines interpersonal, family, and health communication in this emerging intergenerational research area.

More than 13 percent of adult caregivers live more than one hour from their care recipient and 35 percent identified themselves as primary caregivers (AARP, 2009). Though long-distance caregivers lived, on average, a seven-hour drive (nearly 500 miles) from their care recipients, one third visited recipients once a week or more and 50 percent reported spending one day per week providing care while accruing an average of almost $400 per month in travel and care expenses (National Alliance for Caregiving and the Metlife Mature Market Institute, 2004).

Distance adds "unique and complicated challenges to what is already an often emotion-laden and stressful job" and long-distance caregiving is a complex situation that often positions career versus family and creates guilt for the caregiver (NAC/MMMI, 2004: 3). Family members not living close to one another still provide economic aid and support (Stafford, 2005: 14). For example, Kulis (1987) found that, though proximity exerts a strong influence on behaviors such as visits and household assistance, it is not related to parents' and children's feelings and perceptions of each other. Further, geographic distance does not reduce family members' mutual concern for one another (Baldassar et al., 2007) and is not associated with adult child–parent closeness (Lin and Rogerson, 1995). Similarly, elderly individuals' family relationships are emotionally significant even if there is little to no contact with individual family members (Bedford and Blieszner, 2000). Despite this minimal impact on relational quality, research consistently reveals that geographic distance is the strongest predictor of interaction frequency, even after controlling for sex, age, length of residence, marital status, and income (Stafford, 2005).

In a longitudinal study, Kaufman and Uhlenberg (1998) found that, though an increase in distance was positively related to a decline in adult son–mother relationship quality, there was actually a significant relational quality increase for adult daughters with both of their parents. Relatedly, Baldassar and Baldock (2000) found that transnational migrants maintained, and sometimes increased, intimate interactions with close family members years after moving away. Living together or in close proximity is linked to relational dissatisfaction, independence struggles, and interpersonal conflict (Stafford, 2005). Thus, despite the prevailing belief that close proximity is an aspect of strong relational ties because it can provide frequent access to companionship, advice, emotional assistance, or social support, "geographic distance does not pose an insurmountable obstacle to intergenerational relationships" (Stafford, 2005: 65–6).

Engaging in daily living needs such as meal preparation, home maintenance, shopping, providing instrumental support, help around the house or light housekeeping, and personal care to elderly parents does appear to require more proximity (see, e.g., Baldassar et al., 2007; Stafford, 2005). Distant siblings are typically involved in caregiving decisions and tend to provide practical, financial, and emotional support to both their parents and the primary caregivers (Baldassar et al., 2007; Baldock, 2000; Joseph and Hallman, 1998; Litwak and Kulis, 1987).

Interpersonal communication and distance caregiving

Though younger parents are more likely to initiate contact with their distant children, as they grow older and have diminished health, their children become the initiators (Baldassar et al., 2007); in effect, role reversal characteristics in the complex older adult parent–adult child relationship often begin to emerge in this context. According to Aylor (2003), phone calls are the most important type of mediated communication used across long-distance relationships, and also frequently occur in long-distance caregiving (Baldock, 2000). De Wit et al. (1988) identified four hours' drive as the approximate distance where phone contact increased and face-to-face (FtF) contact decreased. Further, Baldassar et al. (2007) noted that distant caregivers provide emotional, financial, and practical care most frequently via phone, letters, email, and texting.

Of course, face-to-face visits are also central in maintaining the long-distance caregiving relationship. This contact is necessary for providing multiple forms of support (Baldassar et al., 2007) and to "take stock" of the parents' living and care situation (Baldock, 2000). One specific form of face-to-face contact for long-distance caregiving is the long-term visit, which ensures a period of intimate contact with the care recipient and provides respite to a primary caregiver, if there is one (Baldassar et al., 2007). Perhaps the most important reason for face-to-face contact between a distant caregiver and a care recipient is for information or instrumental purposes rather than for relational or emotional support (Baldassar et al., 2007; Baldock, 2000).

Distant adult children often feel uninformed about their mothers' care (Schoonover et al., 1988). Distant caregivers attempt to assess a primary caregiver's non-verbal communication, including silence, for hidden cues (Baldassar et al., 2007). Proximal adult children are better able to determine how vulnerable their older adult parents are physically and mentally than children who are distant (Joseph and Hallman, 1998). As such, Baldassar et al. (2007) found that distant caregivers felt they had no right to intervene on decisions made about an elderly parent's care because they were typically absent from the family. NAC/MMMI (2004) also found that long-distance caregivers frequently feel excluded from care decisions made by those who are geographically close.

Information and support from proximal social network members is an important component of both long-distance and intergenerational relationships. Sahlstein (2004) found that long-distance romantic partners engaged in network negotiations as a way to balance spending time together and apart, with these networks serving as relationship-maintaining resources. Further, social networks that include spouses, siblings, friends, neighbors, and the intergenerational parent–child relationship are an integral component of Nussbaum and Fisher's (2009) communication model of competent geriatric medicine delivery. The importance of social network members also thus logically extends to the long-distance caregiver context. Namely, Baldock (1999, 2000) found that distance caregiving involved making arrangements with neighbors or other family members who were proximal to the care recipient. However, elderly parents were sometimes uncomfortable burdening these members of their social networks (Stoller et al., 1992), possibly because they expect their children to care for them regardless of distance (Lee et al., 1995).

End-of-life care

About a century ago death experiences were more common for families because people often died at home with the family involved in care. However, in the twenty-first century, about 80 percent of the 2 million Americans who die each year do so in hospitals (Keeley and Yingling, 2007). Death and dying are taboo topics that most people avoid talking about due to a variety of cultural and social barriers (Keeley and Yingling, 2007; Kreps and Sparks, 2008; Ragan et al., 2008). Approaches to these important issues have evolved over the last few decades, from early preferences to delivery of care provided at home, to the medicalization of bereavement and grief in the 1950s, to a shift back to dying with dignity in one's own home (see Ragan et al., 2008, for detailed discussion).

Researchers have found that the US health-care system often provides inadequate care for the dying (Field and Cassel, 1997; Foley and Gelband, 2001), because many experience diagnosis and treatment issues, particularly when it comes to comfort, pain levels, and psychosocial problems (Bernabei et al., 1998; Martin, Emanuel, and Singer, 2000; Reb, 2003). Effective assessment of pain is important in terms of its control, and information about pain needs to be effectively communicated to providers in order to achieve the balance between adequate pain control and over- or under-medication (Travis and Sparks-Bethea, 2001; Travis, Sparks-Bethea, and Winn, 2000; Panke, 2002). Over-medicating a patient can lead to numerous problems, such as the accumulation of toxins associated with pain medications, renal dysfunction, decreased cognitive functioning, and organ failure. Under-medication can lead to inadequate pain control and unnecessary suffering for the patient.

Although this seems to be improving, dying patients are sometimes treated with a lack of respect, often experiencing miscommunication with providers, while their family members often experience a lack of social support during the end-of-life process (Lawton, 2000). Teno et al. (2004) further indicate that, rather than receiving palliative care benefits, dying Americans are most often offered inadequate pain management, little to no emotional support, and poor communication from the medical providers taking care of them. End-of-life care is often provided by doctors and nurses who have limited training (Barclay et al., 2003; Rhymes, 1990), but this is slowly changing for the better with more attention devoted to palliative and hospice care contexts. In fact, the Obama health-care reform Bill includes a provision that would pay for end-of-life care consultations every five years, giving patients more opportunities to discuss treatment plans that fit with their needs and beliefs (Morrow, 2009). It is certain that relational agency – or fighting for appropriate and effective care – must be employed by caregivers and patients alike during life-threatening illnesses to achieve better health outcomes (O'Hair and Sparks, 2008).

Ragan et al. (2008) describe *palliative care* as encompassing a broader range of patients and services than hospice care, as it typically focuses on the relief of suffering and improvement of quality of life, whereas the goal of *hospice care* is to provide patients and family members with the ability to die at home, surrounded by loved ones. Ragan et al. state that palliative care is often expressed in the following common ways.

- Patients and their families constitute the unit of care (because patients don't suffer in isolation but in a constellation with their families).
- Suffering includes four components: physical, psychological, social, and spiritual.
- Communication is a critical skill in palliative care. (2008: 25)

Researchers have found that emotional support and issues of spirituality are delicate, time-consuming, and challenging aspects of caregiving, often requiring more of a caregiver's time and effort than other daily caregiving tasks (Bakas et al., 2002; Egbert and Parrott, 2003; Egbert et al., 2008; Toseland, Blanchard, and McCallion, 1995). This has been verified by both lay and professional caregivers (Travis and Sparks-Bethea, 2001; Travis, Sparks-Bethea, and Winn, 2000). Caregivers typically serve as the nucleus of support for the needs of patients in end-of-life situations, and, as such, if the caregivers cannot deliver important pain management and psychosocial needs, the patient often suffers (Andrews, 2001), as do close family and friends witnessing the care. Given the uncertainty and worry often connected to accepting one's own death and dying process among people with terminal illnesses, emotional support is also a frequent and essential component of care. Listening to caregiver and patient apprehension, anxiety, and/or fears, and providing kind and thoughtful responses to those in need, is an important aspect of holistic palliative or hospice care. However, this process can be very time-consuming for caregivers, especially when faced with the need to accomplish multiple tasks while providing daily instrumental care to patients (Ragan et al., 2008). Patient irritability and confusion, with aggressive behaviors during late-stage cancer, may make it even more difficult and exhausting for caregivers to provide emotional support. Moreover, both professional and lay caregivers often have little training for providing emotional support, so there is a need for education and training to deal with these issues in order to effectively provide emotional support (Bakas et al., 2002).

Theoretical frameworks informing caregiving and end-of-life contexts

Public health, health intervention, health policy, and health-risk communication scholars increasingly claim that studies must utilize a guiding theoretical framework to generate the type of knowledge needed to create proper and effective evidence-based interventions and ensure their efficacy in helping families. Theories can explain psychological functioning that accounts for the enactment of behavior and behavior change that the intervention is striving to achieve (Michie and Abraham, 2004). Further, theory plays a fundamental role in effecting changes in health-care practice and policy, as well as in patient and provider interaction. Prior research utilized to change policy to improve the nation's health has been under a great amount of scrutiny precisely because of its atheoretical approach (Dean, 1996).

Life-span perspectives of aging and development recognize that individuals are constantly adapting to their environment and that their social interaction is an important part of their ability to adapt across the life course (Baltes, 1987; Baltes and Baltes, 1990; Carstensen, 1991, 1992; Kahn and Antonucci, 1980; Nussbaum, 1989; Pecchioni et al., 2005). Research grounded in life-span developmental perspectives also suggests family bonds play particular roles in this regard. Emotional family interaction may be very important to one's adaptability at various points in life, including the difficult contexts involved in the caregiving experience.

Another important yet often overlooked contextual factor is the caregiver's age or place in the life course. Communication is a developmental phenomenon (Nussbaum et al., 2000, 2002). Individuals communicate differently and have unique communication needs as an aspect of where they are in the life course (Pecchioni et al., 2005). For example, older adults often show more competent communication in comparison to younger adults because they have more life experiences from which to draw. Cohort variability also plays a role. Zietlow and Sillars (1988) state that individuals from different generations who grew up in contrasting sociocultural contexts reveal different communication preferences. Further, Segrin (2003) found that in comparison to older generations, younger people's well-being appears to depend more on receiving social support from diverse sources. These findings are very important for caregivers to consider because the communication channel preferences may vary greatly depending on such variables as age, place in life course, and sociocultural contexts, as well as one's social support network. The risk of not paying attention to such preferences and variations may impact decision-making and overall quality of care.

Other caregiving communication research has examined the use of humor by a family member to cope with the caregiving situation (Sparks-Bethea, Travis, and Pecchioni, 2000) and in parent–adult child discussions of the parent's cancer (Harzold and Sparks, 2007, 2008), how family caregivers coordinate with formal caregivers to administer medications to their care recipients (Travis and Sparks Bethea, 2001; Travis, Sparks-Bethea, and Winn, 2000), and the extent to which adult siblings negotiate parent caregiving (Willyard et al., 2008). Further, Harzold and Sparks (2008) identified the following satisfying communication patterns in older adult parent–adult child discussions of the parent's cancer diagnosis and treatment options: discussing the parent's feelings, the initial diagnosis disclosure, and discussion of treatment procedures. Dissatisfying conversations also involved discussing parental feelings, as well as withholding information from the adult child and discussing the outcome of the cancer (Harzold and Sparks, 2008).

Davidhizar (1999) offered practical suggestions to health-care providers who are asked how to be distant caregivers by adult children, many of which touch upon the interpersonal communication issues described. Adult children should:

1   be aware of how their parents are functioning by taking notice of unusual non-verbal cues and by asking direct questions;
2   keep in mind that it is difficult, discuss parents' needs with them, preferably face-to-face;
3   work to reach consensus about caregiving decisions amongst parents and all adult children;
4   evaluate the existing social network to determine what role they play in parents' lives and consider how formal networks could additionally contribute;
5   actively participate in care management;
6   maintain regular, scheduled contact to provide continuity for the parents and help keep children updated and informed; and
7   make visits count by evaluating the parents' care and visiting doctors with the parents to keep informed.

These suggestions highlight the essential role that communication plays in every aspect of the caregiving process.

Building on suggestions expressed by Bevan and Sparks (2010), communication theory should be employed to understand how caregivers negotiate and communicate care. The study of caregiving is a relatively atheoretical area, though scholars have previously applied equity theory (Ingersoll-Dayton et al., 2003) and cognitive dissonance theory (Lee et al., 1995) with some success, as well as suggesting the potential usefulness of social learning theory (Stoller et al., 1992) and systems theory (Bedford and Blieszner, 2000) to understand caregiving contexts. As Bevan and Sparks (forthcoming) point out, communication theories and theoretical constructs should guide caregiving research toward understanding the varied caregiving contexts from a communication perspective, as well as to instill this research area with more theoretically based scholarship.

For example, Sahlstein (2006b) has examined dialectics and uncertainty, which are viewed as relevant theoretical approaches to long-distance relationships, and this logic can certainly extend to distance caregiving contexts as well (Bevan and Sparks, 2010). Specifically, long-distance partners experience uncertainty so making plans is proposed as a communication practice to impose regularity and structure to the relationship and defend against this uncertainty (Sahlstein, 2006a). Further, failure to meet parental expectations for providing support (Lee et al., 1995) and determining how frequently to travel to care for the elderly parent (Baldock, 1999) can cause their adult children uncertainty and anxiety, suggesting that uncertainty might be relevant in the long-distance caregiver context (Bevan and Sparks, 2010). *The Theory of Motivated Information Management* (Afifi and Weiner, 2004), which Fowler and Fisher (2007) suggested as a useful theoretical framework for understanding family caregiving, focuses on both uncertainty and anxiety, both of which play a huge role in the caregiving experience.

Caregiving is a complex communication environment full of difficult decisions and often unknown stressors. Adult children are frequently torn between moving away to pursue job opportunities and moving near elderly parents to maximize grandparent–grandchild contact (Williams and Nussbaum, 2001). Further, the autonomy-connection dialectic reveals that some caregivers find they did not care about their care recipient but were providing care primarily out of obligation (Baillie, 2007). Because many "sandwich generation" caregivers are often forced to balance work, their own family, and other responsibilities while administering care (NAC/ MMMI, 2004; Schoonover et al., 1988; Wright, Sparks, and O'Hair, 2008), it is not surprising that dialectical tensions exist in this context. The recent application of dialectical theory to intergenerational family communication (Pitts et al., 2009) is also an area of research ripe for further in-depth, systematic examination.

Understanding and encouraging the use of social media

The chapter on social media focuses on the broader influences of social media on the patient and provider interaction, but it is especially important to understand the role of social media in the complex caregiving and end-of-life contexts. For example, technology has been recommended as a method for bridging geographic distance in providing socio-emotional, financial, and informational support (Stoller et al., 1992). Additionally, research indicates that telemedicine, including teleconferencing/ videophone and online support, delivering health services over distances, was viewed as a useful resource for patients, partly because it can connect them with distant family members (Gregg and Whitten, 2003). The notion of teleconferencing has moved beyond the organizational level into family environments. For instance, use of technology has been studied as a link between nursing home residents and their family members, and viewed as fairly successful. Specifically, participants stated that teleconferencing enhanced their interactions, increased satisfaction, and they also revealed an increased tolerance for problems and problem-solving (Mickus and Luz, 2002). Online social networking sites for caregivers, such as ConnectingForCare.com, have developed in recent years, and through these web-based forums, caregivers can communicate helpful information about treatment options and the navigation of the health-care system while also providing emotional support (Jones, 2008). Such new technologies as Skype and Facebook are increasingly becoming available, accessible, inexpensive, and easy, allowing individuals of all skill levels and ages to stay connected.

A more recent study (Demeris et al., 2008) points out that informational technology can alleviate the adult child's stress that accompanies moving parents into a residential facility, particularly when such difficult decisions must be made from a geographic distant caregiver. Specifically, participants who were asked to interact via videophone at least once per week reported appreciating having a sense of closeness, seeing each other's expressions, including the resident in family interactions, and the resident appreciated being able to see new family members or friends, enabling him or her to still feel a part of the family. As such, caregivers could relatively quickly learn to understand illness symptoms, assist in reducing feelings of isolation and loneliness, and easily participate with the entire care team. Overall, all participants were enthusiastic and satisfied, and many participants thought that the videophone improved their communication and efficacy regarding care.

As Bevan and Sparks (forthcoming) reveal, overall findings suggest that identifying and characterizing information-seeking and provision, the types of support, and the nature of non-verbal communication can enhance understanding of how technology can benefit caregiving and end-of-life contexts. Further, focusing on the above issues will also allow public health, medical education, health promotion and health communication scholars to contribute their unique, informed perspectives to caregiving scholarship.

Applying interpersonal conflict research to the caregiving context

Following the ideas of Bevan and Sparks (forthcoming), another interesting way in which interpersonal and health communication scholars can inform the understanding of how individuals negotiate caregiving is in the area of interpersonal conflict. Sahlstein (2006b) noted that little is known about how conflict is managed in long-distance relationships, even though conflict can impact the relationship's stability and satisfaction. Indeed, any aspect of her list of negative qualities in long-distance family relationships are probably relevant and can plausibly give rise to conflict in both caregiver–care recipient and sibling primary–distant caregiver dyads, including:

1 maintenance difficulties, such as expense and inconvenience;
2 tension and stress that arise;
3 difficulty in maintaining current information;
4 difficulty in reassuring, supporting, and comforting each other;
5 low interaction frequency and quantity; and
6 difficulty managing family and individual challenges. (Sahlstein, 2006b)

As Bevan and Sparks (forthcoming) indicate, a number of interpersonal conflict concepts may be relevant to caregiving contexts, including the integrative, distributive, and conflict-avoidance strategies (e.g., Sillars, 1980), and conflict competence (e.g., Canary, Cupach, and Serpe, 2001). Recent research has observed that siblings displayed little consensus regarding who would be the primary caregiver, due to minimal communication about the topic (Connidis and Kemp, 2008), and Baldassar and Baldock (2000) questioned how distant and proximal sibling caregiving negotiations would proceed, suggesting that these conflict concepts are relevant to the study of caregiving as well as to many end-of-life issues. In addition, Pecchioni and Nussbaum's (2001) finding, that mother–daughter discussions prior to dependency mostly involved integrative, solution-oriented conflict strategies that were viewed by participants as fruitful and positive, encourages future study as to how constructive and competent conflict can be beneficial to those involved in caregiving and end-of-life situations.

The notion of serial arguing is also potentially an interesting direction to pursue in future caregiving and end-of-life research (see also Bevan and Sparks, 2010). Serial arguments are ongoing, unresolved sets of conflict episodes that center upon the same issue and have been observed in family relationships across multiple studies (Bevan, Finan, and Kaminsky, 2008; Trapp and Hoff, 1985). The fact that caregiving relationships can be stressful for all involved parties, span many years, and be quite time-intensive creates an environment where serial arguments are particularly likely to develop. Indeed, unresolved rivalry and disagreement regarding their mothers' needs and care characterized distant individuals' relationships with their primary caregiver siblings (Schoonover et al., 1988). Thus, Bevan et al.'s (2008) serial argument process model, which includes important components of serial arguments such as conflict goals, strategies, rumination, and perceived resolvability, might be a useful framework for understanding how serial argument episodes are enacted in caregiving relationships.

Topic avoidance and caregiving/end-of-life

Understanding caregiving and complex end-of-life issues from an interpersonal communication perspective is also likely to involve the notion of topic avoidance. Topic avoidance is a deliberate decision to not share information about a specific topic with a close relational partner (Afifi and Guerrero, 2000) that has been observed in parent–child relationships (e.g., Guerrero and Afifi, 1995) and in multiple relationship contexts that are characterized by a health condition (Bevan, 2009). Communication avoidance has been negatively related to communication satisfaction in intergenerational American and Indian relationships (Giles et al., 2007), and avoidance motivated by a desire to protect oneself has been shown to cause relational dissatisfaction and reduce relational closeness (Dillow, Neary Dunleavy, and Weber, 2009).

Much of the research suggests that all participants in an informal caregiving situation are engaging in topic avoidance regarding care (see, e.g., Bevan and Sparks, 2010). For example, despite the fact that planning for future caregiving can reduce depression and anxiety, many families avoid having this important conversation (Fowler and Fisher, 2007). Further, a caregiver's reported feelings of being uninformed about a parent's care (Schoonover et al., 1988) suggests that the care recipient and other proximal family members continue to avoid the topic of caregiving even as it is occurring. Harzold and Sparks's (2007) finding that a parent's withholding of cancer information from an adult child is dissatisfying also implies that this topic avoidance might be frustrating to caregiving situations in particular. In terms of adult siblings, Willyard et al. (2008) found that, though siblings used avoidance to deal with negotiating who would participate in their parent's care, caregivers also perceived that siblings did little or nothing to assist with caring for parents.

Based upon these findings, focusing on two aspects of topic avoidance might be valuable for studying caregiving situations. First, investigating which participants in the care situation have specific topic avoidance motivations might improve understanding of why individuals are withholding information, with discussion to encourage these individuals to communicate more about caregiving. These topic avoidance motivations include protecting oneself, protecting the relationship, believing the partner will be unresponsive to the topic, believing that there is a lack of closeness with the relational partner, to avoid conflict, and to maintain privacy (Caughlin and Afifi, 2004), which are all reasonable in the caregiving context as well. Second, applying the tenets of Communication Privacy Management (CPM) theory (Petronio, 2002) would assist in understanding the process of topic avoidance in caregiving. CPM's goal is to explain the process of regulating the revealing and concealing of private information via boundaries and privacy rules (Petronio, 2002), making it applicable to understanding how much or how little information may be exchanged among the care recipient or a primary or secondary caregiver (e.g., family members).

In conclusion, caregiving is a unique, complex, often difficult environment that puts unknown stressors on informal as well as formal caregivers involved. Indeed, though caregivers have reported feeling helpless, nervous, frustrated, angry, depressed, drained, worried, and overwhelmed (Schoonover et al., 1988; Stafford, 2005), most do not feel as if they are doing enough for the care recipient (Baldock, 2000) and that they themselves do not need support (Gregg and Whitten, 2003). It is obvious that studying aspects of interpersonal, health, and family communication could substantially reduce the challenges experienced by patients, providers, caregivers, and other care participants. The patient and provider interaction usually includes a caregiver as part of the interactive and decision-making process. Understanding caregiving from a health communication perspective remains an uncharted research territory that we encourage scholars from a variety of theoretical perspectives to explore via interdisciplinary research teams involving complementary communication approaches to care.

Discussion Questions for Caregivers to Improve Care

Caregiving for a loved one, especially caregiving from a distance, can be stressful and challenging. It is important for caregivers to ask these questions to better understand the caregiving situation and provide the best care possible, while also seeking solutions to minimize the burden of providing care.

Is the care recipient receiving proper medical care?

What can be done to improve medical care?

Can the care recipient manage his/her own personal care?

Can the care recipient handle housekeeping and home maintenance tasks?

Can the care recipient move freely and safely in and out of the house?

Can the care recipient make sound decisions?

Are there family members, friends, and/or neighbors who can help?

What community resources are available? Are there co-payments for these services?

What private services are available? What are the costs?

Who will be responsible for which aspects of care?

Discussion Questions for Seeking End-of-Life Care

Decision-making for both the individuals facing a terminal diagnosis and their family members are both difficult and emotional. While communicating about these issues is not always easy, it is important to have these conversations with health-care providers and family members to ensure that end-of-life care satisfies the wishes of the patient. These questions can help to maximize patient comfort and satisfaction in this difficult time.

My doctor informed me that my illness is terminal. What legal matters should I be considering?

Which medical treatments am I willing to consider at this point? What forms do I need to complete so that others know my wishes if I am in a position where I cannot make my desires known?

I know my illness is terminal but I still have unresolved issues with some important people in my life. How can I approach them to talk about my feelings now that I know I am not going to live much longer?

How do I help my family feel better about my diagnosis? My main concern is letting them know I am ready for whatever happens.

How have others with my disease dealt with preparing for death?

Would hospice or palliative care be a good option for me?

PART III

CULTURE AND IDENTITY INFLUENCES ON
PATIENT AND PROVIDER INTERACTION

6 Cultural Characteristics

Case study: the misuse of race in medical diagnosis

I am a 39-year-old Hispanic male born in Stockton, Calif., to a mother who – after many years of unwise eating – has recently been diagnosed with diabetes and to a father I didn't know who floated away at the end of a needle in his sister's garage. I prefer being called Mexican to Hispanic, though I've never been to Mexico. I eat a fat American's diet. Speak American English. Although I don't smoke, I have been living in a big city with polluted air. An American city where I recently was an assistant professor of pediatrics, working in a profession that tries to define my indefinable race without asking for my input.

I helped train medical students and residents who are all taught, as I was when I was a medical student, to assess each patient first in terms of age, race, and gender. Always in that order. A 52-year-old white female, a 3-month-old Asian male, a 39-year-old Hispanic male. The actual identity of patients remains ignored: A 47-year-old African-American female – who's never been to Africa and prefers to call herself black if ever asked by a white doctor, though none ever asks – two-pack-a-day smoker, still living with her mother in South Central Los Angeles, presents with fatigue.

The doctor asks the patient – or the parent of the patient, if you're a pediatrician – for his or her age. The gender is determined during the physical exam. But the doctor usually just assumes the patient's race by looking at the person. My professors told me, and current textbooks still say, that knowing the patient's race helps the doctor make an accurate diagnosis. So the doctor looks at the patient's skin, nose, hair, lips – the silent mouth – and defines ancestry in a single word: Asian, Hispanic, white, African-American. I smiled when one doctor described the Nigerian father of a patient as an African-American. The Nigerian father didn't smile.

The textbooks say that a patient's race can, and should, influence the doctor's thinking about possible diagnoses. An Ashkenazic Jewish baby might have Tay-Sachs disease. A black boy might have sickle cell anemia. A Southeast Asian girl might have thalassemia. Of course, I know that Ashkenazic Jews get Tay-Sachs, but the only baby I ever saw with Tay-Sachs was a Mexican child. I didn't misdiagnose the disease because he was Mexican instead of Jewish.

Do all Hispanics have the same genetic risk for asthma? Do Mexicans and Puerto Ricans eat the same diet? What about a patient from Spain – is he Hispanic in the same way that I am?

My childhood friend Lela wasn't diagnosed with cystic fibrosis until she was 8 years old. Over the years, her doctors had described her as a "2-year-old black female with fever and cough . . . 4-year-old black girl with another pneumonia. Lela is black." Had she been a white child, or had no visible "race" at all, she would probably have gotten the correct diagnosis and treatment much earlier. Only when she was 8 did a radiologist, who had never seen her face to face, notice her chest X-ray and ask, "Who's the kid with CF?"

An emergency-room physician referred a patient to me with this history: "A 14 y.o. black male from South Central LA with a positive tox screen presents with headache. He's probably in a gang." I ordered a CT scan of the patient's head and discovered a large cyst that had blocked the normal flow of cerebral spinal fluid until the fluid had backed up and squashed his brain against his skull. Yes, he had a headache, and he had smoked a joint before going to the hospital.

Those are just two examples of incorrect diagnoses caused by doctors who use racial assumptions to arrive at incorrect medical conclusions. As a physician, such misdiagnoses disturb me. I am also concerned as a father. I am Mexican from California, and my wife is black from Los Angeles. Our daughter is blonde with green eyes and pale skin. I have no known white ancestors, and that kind of heritage – even if it is just a legend – would not be left out of my family's stories. In my wife's case, her mother is now tracing their family's roots back through American history; as of 1843, she has not found a single white ancestor. But my wife's relatives generally have fair skin, and I suspect that my mother-in-law will eventually find a slave owner or overseer or some other white man who is responsible for that, and for my daughter's appearance.

What concerns me is that many years from now, when she is old enough to see a doctor with neither me nor my wife present, the doctor will use what he assumes is her race to misdiagnose her: "A 19-year-old white female presents with irritability."

Here is the crux of the problem: My daughter's race can never be known. Her genetic risk for this or that disease is necessarily imprecise because she is a person, not a race.

Americans used to define anyone who had "one drop of Negro blood" as a Negro, but we now know that definition makes no sense. We learn nothing if we group together as Asian-Americans a man in Seattle who was born in the far eastern portion of the former Soviet Union, a Korean woman living in Toronto, and a child in California with maternal grandparents who immigrated from China and a father whose ancestors came to New Jersey from Europe. There are almost as many definitions of Hispanic as there are Hispanics. Do I have the same genetic risk for sickle cell anemia as a Puerto Rican, a Spaniard, or a Mayan? What about my daughter, and the millions like her in this country, whose racial and ethnic ancestry defies geography and time?

If by using a patient's ancestry in medical discourse we can narrow the range of possible diagnoses, then at least we must be careful to describe accurately the genetic, ethnic, cultural, or geographical variables involved; guessing what category a person fits in is not acceptable. And when "race" cannot possibly matter, let us omit it. What difference does it make if it is an African-American or an Asian who has an earache or ingrown toenail?

Medical-school professors must teach students that a Hispanic is not real. That an Asian-American doesn't exist. That whites exist only in

America: They are Irish in Ireland, Italian in Italy, Spaniards in Spain. That harm – real, physical harm – can come from calling a child with cystic fibrosis an African-American. Race does exist in America, alas. It's why my daughter's history here starts in slavery. It's why my Mexican face identifies me to strangers before they know I'm an educated member of the middle class. It's why nobody dares to ask for details about anybody else's identity.

Richard Garcia, "The misuse of race in medical diagnosis," *The Chronicle of Higher Education* 49 (2003): B15

Although biological differences in race play a role in the incidence of some diseases, a person's cultural background almost always plays a role in the way that health is viewed, received, and discussed (Sparks and Villagran, 2008, 2009; Ojanlatva et al., 1997). We are influenced by a dominant culture or co-cultures: in the broadest sense, the term culture includes who we are as individuals, based on race, ethnicity, gender, age, religious preferences, income, and educational background. And culture, more than any surface unique racial differences, provides a distinctive way to look at and experience the world around us. It is a dynamic force in society. It is a way to express ourselves. It is a way to create ourselves. Culture influences the most fundamental aspects of our existence, such as our assumptions about human nature, the nature of reality, and our relationships to one another and our surroundings (Gudykunst, 1998; Hofstede, 2001; Schein, 1985). Communication is central to this process because language is defined by, reflects, and transmits culture.

Culture is the collective way in which a group of people share and interpret their experiences of the world (Hecht, Jackson, and Pitts, 2005). It defines our socially expected roles (see Stryker, 1987; Thois, 1991), how to competently perform those roles, and the meanings attached to them (Ting-Toomey, 1999). As a result, there is social pressure to conform to the expectations of a social group. Moreover, culture is intergenerationally transmitted, reflecting the values, beliefs, norms, rules, communicative behaviors, and social institutions of a group (Chen and Starosta, 1998). Based on the beliefs and values of our culture, we learn not only the appropriate interaction scripts within our culture, but also the meanings that should be assigned to those interactions (Ting-Toomey, 1999). For example, we learn how to greet strangers, the extent to which older or ill individuals are valued or not, the relationship between our body and our self, as well as our own role within society.

Beliefs and values derived from a cultural group provide a guiding framework for social interaction and help shape expectations for those interactions. It is important to note, however, that cultures are not homogeneous (Gudykunst, 1998). For example, the United States is said to have an "American" culture that focuses on individualism, direct communication, and assumes a low power distance between individuals (Hofstede, 1991; Triandis, 1995). Not everyone living in the US, however, adheres to this dominant style. Co-cultures, also often referred to as sub-cultures, are groups of individuals within a culture whose members share many values with the dominant culture, but also have some values that differ from the larger culture. Most of us belong to multiple co-cultural groups (e.g., age cohorts, health status, gender, and ethnicity) (Al-Deen, 1997; Gudykunst, 1998; Orbe, 1998).

Membership in a co-cultural group shapes our attitudes toward people belonging to dissimilar groups (Allport, 1954; Ting-Toomey, 1999). Membership in a number of co-cultural groups necessitates the management of group boundaries (Ting-Toomey, 1999). For example, when we interact with a person outside of our co-cultural group we identify – usually subconsciously – our similarities and differences (see Tajfel and Turner, 1986). Interacting with others from our same group, then, is comfortable and safe because we know what to expect and do not have to explain or justify our behaviors (Gudykunst, 1995). Interacting with people from other groups, however, may lead to strong emotional reactions as our expectations, based on cultural norms, are violated (Burgoon, 1995; Mackie and Smith, 2002). Individuals tend to think that their own group behaviors are superior and that out-group behaviors are inferior (i.e., in-group bias, Brewer, 1979), resulting in reactions such as "It's just not cool!" Although in- and out-group perspectives are widespread, it is important to note that diverse group perspectives can enhance interactions and minimize group think.

As a consequence of these assumptions about group members, when individuals from different cultural groups communicate, they tend to operate on differing expectations for the interaction. Interactions between such individuals are labeled intercultural communication (Ting-Toomey, 1999). Because all cultures do not have the same underlying beliefs and values, we can compare the expectations of cultures – labeled cross-cultural communication (Ting-Toomey, 1999). An example will help to differentiate intercultural from cross-cultural communication. A physician from a large urban area in the United States (e.g., Los Angeles or Washington, DC) may be seeing a patient who emigrated to the US from a rural area in Mexico. Intercultural aspects of their interaction may include differences in language, social class, age, gender, and socioeconomic status. Cross-cultural aspects of their interaction may be revealed as they discover that each participant has different conceptions about the perceived causes and nature of illness, and different definitions of and values for health and medicine.

As scholars of health communication and aging, Pecchioni and Sparks (2007), argue, it is important to acknowledge the pervasive ageism and racism that exists in the medical profession. For instance, when physicians do not provide older patients with information about clinical trials, even when they think they are acting in the patient's best interests, they are acting on assumptions that may be unfounded. As some empirical evidence shows, older cancer patients fare well in clinical trials when compared to their younger counterparts (see, e.g., Pecchioni et al., 2008). Older patients may well have physical differences from younger patients, but these differences should be established empirically rather than based on limited experience that may be filtered through negative attitudes toward aging (Sparks, 2007). Recent research has also shown that ageism itself can have a toll on health, since patients who believe in negative age stereotypes early in life are more likely to suffer worse health effects later on (Levy et al., 2009). Think about how often you have heard a statement such as: "She is so young to have that terrible disease." Such statements suggest that it is acceptable, even expected, for older people to suffer from disease. Co-cultural differences based on ethnicity, race, or nationality may be even more pervasive in health care than ageism as differences extend across the spectrum of care. Ethnic minorities have less access to health care, report lower levels of trust in health-care professionals, delay going to doctors for tests, and are less likely to be offered high-quality care options with cutting-edge technology (Nelson, 2002). This broad spectrum of variable health-care access makes the health-care experience quite different, depending on one's co-cultural group, at least in the United States.

Culturally related communication barriers, stereotyping, and biases all get in the way of effective communication and subsequent decision-making regarding diagnostic tests, treatment options, and the like because of confusion and fear about the health-care system itself, providers within the system, and medical language (Van Servellen, 2009). The magnitude of health-disparity issues has been widely disseminated through an Institute of Medicine review titled, "Unequal Treatment: Confronting Racial and Ethnic Disparities in Health Care" (IOM, 2002b). The Report explores the underpinnings of health disparities and health care in terms of the extent to which underserved minorities receive lower-quality health care than non-minorities. Communication contributes to these health disparities due to a lack of culturally and linguistically appropriate messages about cancer, especially since communicative and behavioral practices of Latino patients do not necessarily coincide with a biomedical approach to treatment and prevention (Collins, Villagran, and Sparks, 2008; Cora-Bramble and Williams, 2000; Kreps, 2006; Office of Minority Health, 2005; Villagran and Hoffman, 2008). Culturally competent communicators (including both patients and providers) can reduce such disparities by practicing awareness and mindfulness during each and every medical encounter.

Often the individuals most in need of interventions are those who are the hardest to reach or who have the fewest resources. Overall, ethnic minorities, low-income populations, and individuals with low health literacy do not have equal access to the relevant information necessary to navigate the health-care system and obtain optimal care (Fiscella et al., 2000). Evidence suggests that information is more likely to be retained when messages are tailored and timed to coincide with patients' needs and skills (Bandura, 1997).

Race, socioeconomic status, education, and literacy clearly affect health outcomes and disparities in care (Kutner et al., 2006). The Office of Disease Prevention and Health Promotion (2006) Report emphasizes the need to clearly identify causal factors for disparities in care so that interventions are developed to remediate these factors. There is growing evidence concerning the mediational roles that health disparities play in the access to and utilization of health care. General patient barriers to obtaining information include psychological adjustment to diagnosis and treatment, (Sparks and Turner, 2008), cultural differences, (Collins, Villagran, and Sparks, 2008), communication with providers (e.g., Sparks and Villagran, 2008), age differences (Sparks and Nussbaum, 2008), coping styles and emotion (Sparks and Turner, 2008), and low literacy (Kreps and Sparks, 2008).

In terms of the relationship between culture and patient–provider interactions, culture shapes values and beliefs about health, expectations for every visit to a care provider, knowledge, attitudes, and ability to operate within the health-care system. Culturally appropriate messages are more effective than non-culture specific messages at gaining the attention, stimulating information processing, and promoting health behavior change for patients (Krueter and Haughton, 2006). Culture permeates every part of our world and therefore also has a pervasive impact on the health-care process. Personal cultural orientations, local culture, regional culture, and national culture all impact health care because they frame the policies and procedures of the health-care system, and they shape the way in which health communication occurs. For providers, patients, and caregivers, culture creates a context for communication and a set of rules or norms about how that communication will occur.

Culture is also the framework by which members of a community construct and explain health-related problems. Experiences are defined within the culture of the patient, based on a constructed meaning for each health-care interaction (Dutta-Bergman, 2004). Each medical encounter is situated within a culture, and culture is created and experienced among individuals, communities, and societies; each of these levels of culture contribute uniquely to the way providers and patients interact. The following are examples of these.

- Individuals: Each patient and each provider brings his or her own cultural lens to the medical encounter. This level is the most fundamental and obvious place where culture comes into play because each interaction is created and interpreted based on individuals' awareness, knowledge, attitudes, self-efficacy, skills, and commitment to dyadic communication and shared decision-making. Patients make individual health choices, and choose whether or not to be involved in their own care.
- Groups: The patient's family and other caregivers typically share the cultural background of the patient that plays an important role in the provider–patient interaction. Family members can also be instrumental in questioning how a patient's health-care choices support or conflict with their cultural values. For example, when a provider recommends that a newborn should not be circumcised, or that a teenage girl should receive an HPV vaccination, or that a terminally ill patient should be taken off life support, the family as a group decision-making body will make their decision in part based on their cultural views. In these examples, the patient and physician are not the only two people involved in a

health-care decision, but, rather, the patient is an agent or representative of their family group.

A patient's orientation toward the importance of group identification versus personal needs is an example of the individualism–collectivism construct (Hofstede, 2001). Specifically, collectivistic cultures that emphasize the importance of group affiliation typically discourage assertive behaviors that can foster agency and a collaborative relationship with a physician (Kim et al., 2000). More individualistic patients may be less constrained by their group affiliations when talking with providers (Kim et al., 2000). In contrast, members of collectivist cultures may place greater emphasis on the needs of the family instead of the needs of the patient, thus diminishing the likelihood of undertaking costly or difficult treatment regimes.

- Organizations: Health organizations such as insurance companies and hospitals create rules for their members, provide support for health communication programs, and make policy changes that encourage or require specific action in the medical encounter (Villagran and Hoffman, 2008). Organizations are sometimes affiliated with a specific religious or cultural group, and are often responsible for enacting cultural values of their sponsoring religion or culture. For example, even though abortion is legal in the US, providers and patients at Catholic hospitals do not typically have the option to terminate an unwanted pregnancy because the Catholic Church opposes abortion. Also, Muslim law prohibits autopsy since bodies are supposed to be buried immediately. Muslim patients who require an autopsy for legal reasons, therefore, may not be handled according to this cultural norm if the organization is not familiar with customs that differ from traditional US health-care procedures. Even something as simple as a revealing hospital gown required by a provider can prevent some Muslim women visiting the doctor. Muslim women who are patients may feel humiliated, in part because they are compelled to sit in waiting rooms while wearing drafty paper gowns. The provider may not even see the patient if she leaves, or fails to even show up for a surgical procedure, to avoid such a situation.
- Communities: Community opinion leaders and policymakers can be instrumental in facilitating culturally sensitive health-care interactions between providers and patients in their area. Providers deliver their services in a community that can hinder or support, either in part or in full, their actions and the actions of their patients. Community channels of information have the capacity to change patients' attitudes and beliefs, and can also provide support for culturally sensitive medical interactions. For example, communities where environmental hazards cause health problems for residents can work to equip providers with information about the hazard. Providers can then work together with community leaders to relay culturally appropriate messages to their patients. If a community with a large older adult population has an air pollution problem, community leaders can provide doctors with accurate information about the hazard to help them treat patients with

breathing issues. Channels of information appropriate for older adults can also be used to reinforce providers' recommendations after the medical encounter.

Culture-centered perspective of health communication

The culture-centered approach to health communication offers a lens for analyzing and interpreting data from marginalized members of minority populations (Dutta, 2008). Dutta-Bergman's (2004) cultural perspective serves as a framework to begin developing shared meanings about health experiences and grounded theories about ideological and power differences. The cultural approach is appropriate for research on cultural issues in health care because it helps examine structure and culture as the core of health communication processes and behaviors. Since minority populations tend to be limited by structural issues such as lack of basic resources, including information, these structural issues have the potential to explain the reflexive nature of health-related human behavior and communication. It should be noted that, even though structure and culture may help explain communication and behavior, this does not guarantee that people will respond to these issues consistently.

Dutta (2008) suggests that polymorphism is an important aspect of the cultural framework that allows researchers to explore how members of a community use communication to negotiate multiple meanings of events. Polymorphism refers to the notion that a patient and a provider may have two different views of reality, and both versions can coexist to shape the health-care interaction. Sometimes the obvious way to resolve differing views of health care is just to let go of your own perceptions of a situation in favor of the perceptions of another person. In contrast to this, polymorphism suggests seeking complementary ways to allow alternative views to work together in the medical encounter (Dutta, 2008). If a provider and patient come from two different cultures, for example, each may have his or her own views of how to treat a recurrent health problem. The provider may favor a more biomedical approach, such as prescribed medication or surgery. The patient may prefer alternative treatments, such as meditation or acupuncture. A polymorphic approach to this dilemma would mean that the patient and provider would work together to communicate their feelings and come up with a mutually satisfying plan of action. The treatment could then include acupuncture, yoga, and prescription medication, and thus validate multiple approaches to the issue. Polymorphism opens the door to looking at communication for dialectical tensions that the members of a cultural community must negotiate.

At the heart of the culture-centered framework for health communication is the goal of raising the level of agency for the members of the minority population (Dutta-Bergman, 2004). In this model, experiences are defined within the culture of the patient, based on a constructed meaning for each health-care interaction (Dutta-Bergman). From a culture-centered perspective, choice would be tempered by perceptions of social and political constraints, based on the cultural interpretation and construction of meaning. O'Hair et al. (2003) point out that the patient's level of agency is "often restricted and undermined by institutional and social forces" (p. 198). These "institutional and social forces" are the ideologies present in the health-care setting. Research on patients' experiences in communicating with providers reveals themes of control, power, and patient resources (Ellison and Buzzanell, 1999; Gibbs and Franks, 2002) that fit in with the O'Hair et al. (2003) model. Moreover, in their research conceptualizing patients' satisfaction with providers, Ellingson and Buzzanell (1999) link surface themes such as physicians' amount of respect, care, and reassurance of expertise with root themes of power and control, thus contextualizing the medical encounter within a particular cultural perspective.

Hippocrates argued that it should be the physicians' responsibility to determine the level of information patients should receive about their condition or diagnosis (Gillotti and Applegate, 2000). Contrary to this approach, a culture-centered view of health-care highlights the voices of minority populations as a central force in health-care decision-making. In this manner, culture "is conceptualized as both transformative and constitutive, providing an axis for theorizing the discursive processes through which meanings are socially constructed" (Dutta-Bergman, 2004: 241).

Cultural issues and the structure of health care

According to the culture-centered approach to health communication, marginalization of cultural minorities results in fewer resources and opportunities for participation in health care due to structural forces (Dutta, 2008). The structure of health care is one factor that contributes to social and political disparities for racial and ethnic minorities (Kreps, 2006). The National Center of Minority Health and Health Disparities (NCMHD) (2009) defines health disparities as "differences in the incidence, prevalence, mortality, and burden of diseases and other adverse health conditions that exist among specific population groups in the United States." While some research links health disparities to socio-demographic characteristics of minority patients, other researchers demonstrate that racial and ethnic disparities exist even when patients' ages, income levels, insurance status, and severity of medical condition are consistent (Office of Minority Health, 2005). The next section outlines differences in health care based on cultural factors that impact provider–patient interactions.

Ethnic differences in the medical encounter

Even though culture has a significant impact on provider–patient interactions, the exact nature of how culture shapes health care is not completely known (Rosenberg et al., 2006). Studies have shown that there are considerable disparities in terms of access to health care, and in health outcomes for patients who are from racial and ethnic minorities; 48 percent of health-care providers in the United States treat 82 percent of all minority patients, making it difficult for these providers to spend adequate time with each patient (The Commonwealth Fund, 2009). Health organizations are less likely to provide clinically necessary and routine procedures for minorities, and are more likely to deliver low-quality health services to these patients (Smedley, Stith, and Nelson, 2003). Health-care disparities have been linked to patients' knowledge levels, attitudes, organizational factors in the health-care system, and cultural and social values (Thomas, Fine, and Ibrahim, 2004). Research indicates that intercultural medical encounters often result in less satisfaction and more miscommunication than interactions between a patient and provider from the same culture (Harmsen et al., 2003).

In terms of providers' communication with minority patients, there are several significant findings. First, some studies indicated that physicians exhibit less empathy and emotion toward minority patients, although these findings seem to be mixed (Cooper et al., 2003). Physicians tend to offer more detailed medical explanations and interviews with non-minority patients, and allow their non-minority patients to ask more questions (Shapiro and Saltzer, 1981). As a result, some intercultural medical interactions never achieve shared understanding between the patient and provider (Cass et al., 2002). In the US, Blacks, Hispanics, and Asians are also more likely than Whites to view communication from providers as disrespectful toward them based on their ethnic background, and most minority patients believe they would have received better medical care if they belonged to a different racial group (Johnson et al., 2004b). Black patients tend to mistrust providers more often (Stroman, 2000), and providers are also more likely to misinterpret communication of ethnically diverse patients because of lack of knowledge about cultural differences in communication styles (Banks, Ge, and Baker, 1991).

Finally, ethnic minority patients are also less likely to receive referrals for certain treatments than non-minority patients (Ibrahim et al. 2003; Rucker-Whitaker, Feinglass, and Pearce, 2003). Reasons for these disparities may be rooted in providers' perceptions about potential transportation and economic barriers associated with visiting a specialist who may not practice near the homes of their economically disadvantaged and/or non-White patients (Kinchen et al., 2004). Conversely, providers who are members of minority groups and who routinely see minority patients tend to be more attuned to issues such as cultural sensitivity, flexibility in financial arrangements for patients, and the needs of vulnerable populations when making referrals (Kinchen et al., 2004).

Issues such as language barriers and specific cultural values have a potential impact on the way patients experience and communicate about health care. Patients who are members of ethnic or racial minority groups are less likely to be assertive or engage in social talk with providers from dominant cultural groups, and less likely to discuss their concerns, symptoms, feelings, or expectations for the medical encounter (Johnson et al., 2004a; Rivadeneyra et al., 2000). Minority patients who are more educated may communicate more with providers than less-educated ethnic and racial minority patients (Sleath, Rubin, and Wurst, 2003). A major factor in diminished interaction in medical encounters by minority members is a lack of skill level or confidence in speaking with providers in a non-native language.

Language

Language is one of the most critical barriers to quality health care for doctors and patients belonging to different ethnic and cultural groups (Jacobs et al., 2003). Language barriers impede access to health organizations, diminish the potential quality of health-care services, and increase the risk of unintended health outcomes due to miscommunication (Flores, 2005; Smith, 2009). Since English is the most common language in the US, most providers conduct medical interviews in English. Limited English Proficiency (LEP) is defined as "a limited ability to listen, speak, read, and write in English, and speak[ing] English less than 'very well'" (Shin and Bruno, 2003). Non-concordance occurs when a patient and provider do not share a common primary language. When LEP patients visit English-speaking doctors, miscommunication can often occur (Gany et al., 2007).

Language barriers serve as a major obstacle for many patient–provider interactions because approximately 47 million persons in the United States speak a language other than English at home, and at least 22 million persons in the US have LEP (Shin and Bruno, 2003). Although some regions do have more residents with LEP than others, 46 states experienced an increase in their LEP populations between 1990 and 2000 (Shin and Bruno, 2003). In some regions, LEP patients speak a common language such as Spanish, but in many urban areas providers and hospitals see patients whose primary languages range from Vietnamese to Swahili to Maori.

Research suggests there are substantial differences in the amount of patients' question-asking between language-concordant and language-discordant consultations (Seijo, Gomez, and Freidenberg, 1991). In addition to problems interacting with providers, language barriers for non-English-speaking patients might include making appointments, locating appropriate health-care facilities, reading signage in provider offices, completing patient intake forms, and reading prescription and drug interaction information. When seeking health care, patients with LEP often have worse access to care and lower satisfaction levels compared with English speakers (Gany et al., 2007). Linguistic barriers can lead to patient non-compliance, dissatisfaction, poor perceptions of quality of care (Ramirez, 2003; Sleath and Rubin, 2002). Seijo et al. (1991) suggest that non-concordant language may also have an impact on physicians' communicative behaviors in medical interactions. Physicians make cultural judgments about patients based on the language the patient speaks, and based on their appearance (Perloff et al., 2006).

Although Title VI of the Civil Rights Act requires US medical facilities to provide translators for patients with limited English proficiency, translators are not typically involved in every aspect of patient care and decision-making, and many are poorly trained or inexperienced with translating medical information (Ku and Flores, 2005). In some cases, family members will attend doctor visits with their parents and act as translators (McGorry, 1999). Even though their language skills allow them to speak in both English and the patient's native language, the family member is not typically experienced with using specific medical jargon, or detailing treatment options and drug protocols. If the translating family member has never heard of a word used by a provider, they may not be able to properly translate that word to their own language. In addition, direct translation does not always convey the intended meaning of the words so the same combination of words in two different languages may not produce the same meaning. For example, cancer terms such as "yearly," "mammogram," "diagnosed," "risk factors," "at risk," and "cancer" mean different things to English and Spanish speakers.

Even when the provider and patient share a primary language, regional or national differences in the use of that language can impact the meaning of communication (Villagran and Lucke, 2005). For example, a word or phrase that means one thing to someone from Spain may not mean the same thing to someone from Mexico or Argentina. Similarly, terminology related to cancer care in Britain may be totally different from terms used in the US, even though English is the primary language in both countries. In addition to the actual words spoken by patients and providers, the way the words are used provide clues to their meaning. These nuances are culturally bound. That is, choices to say or not say certain things and the stress put on certain words or syllables can change the meaning of a message. Someone not fluent in a language can miss the prescribed meaning of a message even though they believe they understood what the other person said. Even when the patient and provider are generally concordant, they may have differences in language use that create an opportunity for miscommunication to occur.

Another important issue related to culture and language in medical encounters is that family members who translate information may be barriers to open communication between patients and providers. For example, women from some cultures are less likely to share personal information about their symptoms with their provider if their child is asked to act as the translator. An adult child who attends a doctor visit with their LEP parent or grandparent might communicate directly with the physician in an effort to conceal a negative diagnosis from the patient. If the LEP patient does not understand the English conversation, he or she may not get a full account of his or her own medical situation. For instance, a study in Japan revealed that although their family members were told about their loved one's condition and prognosis, less than 25 percent of cancer patients were told that they had cancer before they died of the disease (Aoki et al., 1997). The will of the family was taken to reflect the will of the patient, so the family made treatment decisions and withheld information about the cancer to allow the patient less psychological distress.

The LEP patient relies on the family member to translate important information, but if this does not occur the provider may be unaware that the patient did not receive important information. In the United States, withholding medical information from a patient goes directly against the standard rules about informed consent from patients about their own treatments. A patient cannot make informed choices about care options unless he or she is aware of his or her diagnosis. Family member translators have the ability to reveal or conceal important information from the patient, so if they do not translate this information, in effect they take away a patient's right to be aware of his or her diagnosis. Professionally trained medical interpreters can help with language barriers, and research shows that the use of professional interpreters decreases costs and reduces misdiagnosis (Smith, 2009).

Fatalism

Fatalism can be defined as a belief in the statement "If someone is meant to get cancer, they will." Fatalistic views of illness stem from cultural, racial, ethnic, religious, educational, and/or socioeconomic differences among patient populations. Minority members who have a strong sense of fatalism are more likely to feel anxiety and psychological distress about illness (Villagran, Collins, and Garza, 2008; Ross, Mirowski, and Cockerham, 1983) than patients who do not believe in fatalism. They are also less likely to comply with treatment recommendations by providers or to seek treatment for themselves or their families (Baquet and Hunter, 1995).

Although fatalistic views based on religion can offer a sense of hope for patients and their families, religious convictions can also lead to a belief that God, or some other higher power, ultimately controls whether or not a person gets well. For example, strong religious beliefs lead minority patients to believe illnesses are predetermined by God, and should therefore be accepted or endured in accordance with God's will (Sabogal et al., 1987). In these cases, the patient and his or her family may also view treatments as being only as effective as God's plan for the patient will allow. Sometimes this belief means patients will not comply with providers' treatment recommendations or seek treatment for themselves or their families. In other cases, a patient may not believe the illness is the work of God but rather a result of behaviors not in line with the will of God. The Good God perspective relates to the idea that God is the healer who can take away the illness caused by bad behavior or a lack of balance in a person's life (Villagran et al., 2008).

Gender roles

Gender norms are closely tied to culture, so cross-cultural communication between men and women from different cultures may be difficult unless both parties understand the cultural influence of gender on communication processes. The World Health Organization (2009) states that gender is a powerful social determinant of health that interacts with other important factors such as a patient's age, family structure, income, education, and social support.

Sex is the term used for biological differences, while gender is the term to differentiate between traditional roles of men and women based on culture. Although it is often believed that biology determines differences between men and women, for example, in cancer incidence and mortality rates (e.g., that women are more likely to develop breast cancer than men), gender differences are also important. One instance of how gender impacts cancer is that of lung cancer. Although men are statistically more likely to get lung cancer, some of the reasons for this fact are based in gender issues. Men are more likely to work in occupations that expose them to occupational lung carcinogens, such as insecticides, pesticides and diesel. Men are also less likely to smoke low-tar/nicotine brands that might be viewed as "women's cigarettes" because of their thinner shape, or because they are marketed to women. Women however, may inhale more deeply on cigarettes because the smaller, thinner brands require a stronger inhalation. Women are also more likely to choose to smoke as a means to reduce their weight, because there are stronger social pressures on women than on men to be thin. All of these differences in potential causes of lung cancer can be traced to gender norms that are culturally constructed.

There is a significant stigma associated with illness in some cultures (Yang et al., 2007), and stigma tends to vary based on cultural views about gender. In all cultures, questions about maintaining sexuality and gender roles often come up when a person is diagnosed with serious illness. For example, patients with sexually transmitted diseases or cancer may be perceived as less attractive, or even as "damaged" or undesirable. Sometimes stigmatized views of illness occur because of cultural misperceptions about the nature of a particular disease. In some cultures, for example, a cancer diagnosis is seen as a sign that a person lives an unbalanced or unhealthy lifestyle. HIV/AIDS has different stigma for women versus men in many cultures (Parker and Aggleton, 2003), and communication with providers is shaped by the patient's cultural view of his or her condition. A lack of information about the exact causes of cancer may lead to inappropriate stigma for persons with certain conditions because others may think the reason they are sick is that they did something wrong, or are being punished. Patients who experience discrimination because of cultural misperceptions about illness suffer two tragedies – the unfair discrimination, and the illness itself.

Power

Certain cultures place great emphasis on a sense of respect for persons in positions of power. Consider how much perceptions of power impact the way we communicate with others. Although a doctor is likely to tell a patient, "Now I want you to make an appointment to see me again if you feel any more pain," it is unlikely that the patient would respond, "Now next time I come for an appointment, I don't want you to leave me waiting for over an hour to see you." Even though the exchange seems honest and clear, the first example would be viewed as a reasonable instruction, while the second statement would seem inappropriate. The reason for this distinction is the power difference between the patient and the provider. Power is a cultural issue, and it differs based on the cultural context within which communication occurs.

Culturally based power difference between patients and providers may lead to several undesired outcomes for patients and their families. First, patients from cultures that place a great emphasis on status may ask fewer questions of their physicians in medical interviews because the patient is concerned about challenging the doctor's authority (see, e.g., Collins, Villagran, and Sparks, 2008). For example, Latino patients may be very agreeable and accept what a doctor says without question due to the Latino culture and its emphasis on respect (Carbone et al., 2007). Based on cultural perceptions about the power of providers, it should not be assumed that all patients desire to be active participants in decisions about their health (Charles et al., 2005).

Some research further suggests that patients from Korean and Mexican cultural backgrounds have less need for information and shared decision-making than non-minority White American patients (Blackhall et al., 1995). Even when patients do want more information from their provider, minority patients and their families may resist asking difficult questions, or questions they think might be viewed as trivial or unimportant. Providers who desire to minimize power differences must anticipate the information needs of minority patients and interact in the expected manner.

Conclusion

As Pecchioni et al. (2008) point out, it is important to acknowledge that patients are not all the same in terms of ethnicity, age, and so on. This acknowledgment should extend not just to the physical realm. Most health-care professionals continue to operate based on the biomedical model of health and illness, in which the body is treated as a machine in isolation from its environment. The biopsychosocial model, however, provides us with a broader lens for examining patients' responses to illness because it acknowledges that individuals operate within a web of individual and social roles. Conrad (1987) proposed the use of "disease" to refer to the physical ailment and "illness" to refer to the social elements of the disease. Thus, an individual is not his or her diagnosis, but makes sense of that diagnosis within a web of cultural expectations. In this perspective, then, health-care personnel must identify each patient's attitudes toward the causes of illness and treatment options, definitions of quality of life, availability of social support and the like. The body is no longer a machine, but a living organism in communication with its physical and cultural environments.

Improving communication is central in efforts to reduce cancer health disparities, or significant differences in the overall rates of disease and/ or death among members of specific cultural groups, as compared to the health status of the general population. These differences occur in part because of biases, stereotyping, prejudice, and most importantly because of a lack of communication about health issues among certain groups. Reducing disparities is directly related to understanding how culture impacts our health-related attitudes, beliefs, and behaviors. This means not only gaining a clearer understanding of the impact of culture on patients, but also how cultures play a role in communication among health providers and health organizations responsible for the delivery of medical services.

Discussion Questions to Minimize Cultural Barriers

Cultural differences can influence the communication between patients and providers, and have the potential to cause misunderstandings and patient non-adherence to prescribed treatments. However, with greater awareness of cultural differences, these barriers can be minimized. Patients and providers can ask themselves questions, such as the following, to better understand how to effectively communicate with an individual of a different cultural background.

How is the patient's/provider's culture different from my own culture?

What aspects of that culture might influence the way he/she communicates?

What aspects of my own culture influence my communication?

How does he/she communicate non-verbally? What can I learn from these non-verbal cues?

How can I express my cultural needs clearly and concisely?

7 Social Identity

Wendy Balazik was a young, physically fit woman who enjoyed running, hiking, and music. She worked at a non-profit organization, and attended graduate school in communication. In class, Wendy was always the person her classmates counted on to deliver the funny question or witty comment when a lecture had become too boring. She was smart, articulate, and interesting. One additional piece of information is that despite never smoking cigarettes, Wendy was diagnosed with stage-four lung cancer that spread to her brain. The fact that she has cancer should not be the first thing you know about Wendy because her cancer did not define who she was as a person. She was still the same woman before and after her diagnosis, except that she had to learn first hand how to communicate about terminal illness with doctors and caregivers.

Before her death in April 2009, Wendy was kind enough to share her thoughts on how her strong sense of identity helped shape her approach to cancer. "I have always been taken to the doctor by my mother and I am very comfortable going to the doctor so for me it was not that much of a problem, and I am rather outgoing so I try not to get intimidated by doctors. I started with a small cough and I thought I was just tired from school, so I went in to the doctor. If I hadn't gone in to find out what was going on I never would have known. I would just encourage people to take control of their situation by going to the doctor because if you don't know you can't take control of it. Especially with your own health, it is much worse to not know what's going on than to know and be able to do the best you can to fix it . . . Owning it makes you less scared."

Wendy also felt fortunate to have doctors who were very good communicators. "She (the doctor) had my X-ray up across the room and I could see that something was weird with my lungs – especially the big white blob-looking thing at the bottom of my left lung. She put her hand on my knee and said she saw what could be cancer . . . She tried to calm me down and she was wonderful.

"Then I was sitting with the oncologist who actually confirmed that it was cancer. I was sitting on the doctor's table and instead of leaning over, or towering over me to talk, he actually leaned back against the cabinet so we were at eye level. He looked right at me as he spoke to me. I guess that is part of the reason he made me feel comfortable because he looked right at me and I could tell he was assessing the situation as we were talking. I think he was trying to assess my education level (and my friend's) to see how to handle things. It may have only taken him like two minutes, but he paused and spoke directly to my friend and me. He didn't talk over me, and he didn't talk down at me, he just talked to us like people. He said I'm not going to tell you anything worse than it is, and I'm not going to tell you anything better than it is . . . I really felt he brought his 'A game' to the interaction."

Wendy discussed the way her doctor connects with her by viewing her as a person, instead of a set of numbers in a chart. "I feel like it is more of a partnership than just me taking orders from a doctor. For me, what matters is that my doctor remembers personal things about me and he seems to be talking to me . . . He also gave me his email address and when I emailed him he responded in less than seven minutes. I hope he wasn't responding on his BlackBerry while he was sitting in traffic!"

Finally, Wendy shared her thoughts about how a young person should talk to a friend with terminal illness. "My friends have cried with me, and I have cried, but I don't want to sit around and have 'Wendy pity parties' all the time. In other words, I don't want to always be sad and just talk about cancer all the time. I just want to talk about normal everyday things in my life like my friends and their relationships, their days at work, cool restaurants and shops. It's not a denial thing but it's not all about me and my cancer, all of the time. That is the best way to help me when they talk to me." Wendy Balazik had a strong social identity that was built from the facts that were most important to who she was and wanted to be – a proud daughter, friend, woman, activist, athlete, and student. Cancer never defined her; it only denied her the opportunity to live longer.

If social identity is formed by the collection of group memberships that define an individual, probably no one would want to include being a terminally ill patient in their social identity collection. Patients who are diagnosed with a chronic or terminal disease gain membership in a group of people who share a common set of symptoms, side-effects, and challenges in dealing with providers. Barriers faced by groups of patients who deal with similar physical and psychological issues can have a major impact on self-concept (Williams, 2008). For example, after a negative diagnosis some patients immediately begin to question their own identity with thoughts of biological degradation ("How could my body do this to me?"), to destiny ("Will I possibly be able to get through this?"), to transformations in self ("Losing my breast to cancer makes me feel that I'm no longer a woman") (Villagran, Fox, and O'Hair, 2007). Although illness is never a positive development in a person's life, the way illness is experienced is based in part on the patient's pre-diagnosis identity.

Shifts in social identity and health can have particular effects on medical decision-making in the doctor–patient relationship. Through communicating with others, patients diagnosed with an illness often see themselves differently and start to recognize that others may view them differently as well (see Harwood and Sparks, 2003; Sparks and Harwood, 2008; Villagran et al., 2007). Some patients will take on an active role in their own care by focusing on the goals of treatment as a process. Other patients might try to avoid dealing with illness through denial, or by refusing to follow their doctor's advice. Some patients even become depressed and therefore lose the ability to be fully involved in the care process in an assertive manner. If a patient feels he or she just does not want to be labeled with illness, then denial is more likely to occur. A young person, for example, who gets diagnosed with asthma, might choose to deny her diagnosis because accepting it would mean she would be labeled as "sick" or "chronically ill" for the rest of her life. If, instead, the patient chooses to attribute her symptoms to seasonal dust in her environment, or a cold, she can avoid the permanent change in her identity and avoid group membership among asthmatic patients.

The reality for most doctors and patients is that the fear, dread, and terror that accompany certain diagnoses require a greater emphasis on communication processes to combat negative assessments of self. Open, honest communication with providers can be a valuable weapon against the assault on self-identity that is perpetuated by a negative diagnosis. Communication becomes more important as cognitive, affective, and behavioral responses to illness combine with biological problems that the patient strives to overcome. In this chapter, we introduce a framework for examining how social identity is impacted by illness. We will specifically examine identity shifts that may occur based on illness and how these identity shifts frame interactions between providers and patients.

Social identity theory

Social identity theory (SIT: Tajfel and Turner, 1986; see also Harwood and Giles, 2005) explains individual responses to difficult situations based on group memberships. In recent years, SIT has been applied to the health communication literature (see, e.g., Villagran, Wittenberg-Lyles, and Hajek, 2007; Harwood and Sparks, 2003; Sparks and Harwood, 2008; Sparks and Villagran, 2008, 2009; Villagran and Sparks, 2010; Villagran, Sparks, and O'Hair, 2007), with specific attention to issues of identity based on the diagnosis, treatment, and recovery from serious illnesses such as cancer. SIT is a broad socio-psychologically grounded theory of intergroup relations that highlights the importance people ascribe to their identities, the ways in which they protect them, and the ways in which they respond when their identities are threatened (Shinnar, 2008).

SIT helps us understand how people are motivated to maintain a positive view of themselves by identifying with groups they perceive to be desirable, and then comparing themselves and other in-group members to another set of people who are perceived to be out-group members. For example, a person might view himself as young, or a member of the younger generation, and would then perceive the young generation as the in-group. Being a member of the younger generation would be viewed as more desirable than being a member of the older generation, or "old people," who are perceived to be an out-group. SIT generally centers on identification with large social groups such as age, culture, sexuality, and so on, but can also be applied to smaller and more specialized groups, including an organizational group, a family, or even a particular disease condition. Table 7.1 lists some of the most common social groups that create our social identities in everyday life.

Social identity is directly related to patient–provider relationships

Table 7.1 Aspects of identity

Level of communication	Basis of group identity
Intrapersonal identities	Personality traits
	Emotional needs
	Consciousness
	Self-concept
Interpersonal identities	Intimate relationship status
	Friendships
	Interpersonal relationships
	Co-worker relationships
	Computer-mediated relationships
Socio-cultural identities	Gender
	Ethnicity
	Age
	Nationality
	Sexual orientation
	Talents and abilities
	Social status
	Education level

Source: Adapted from Richey (2003); Villagran, Fox, and O'Hair (2007)

because we use our social identity to help us deal with difficult situations such as illness. For example, when a patient sees herself as intelligent and educated, she is more likely to engage in shared decision-making with her provider (Villagran et al., 2007). On the other hand, negative social identity can emerge when a patient perceives her group membership to be threatened or less desirable than other group memberships (Shinnar, 2008). An African-American patient, for example, may have a perception that her ethnic identity puts her in jeopardy of receiving sub-standard care because of discrimination by her provider (Williams, Neighbors, and Jackson, 2008). The patient views her ability to interact with a provider and receive high-quality health care based on the groups to which she belongs. Ethnic identity, level of education, age, and identification with a whole host of other social groups may have a positive or negative impact on health interactions because we choose whether or how to communicate with our providers based on the perceived significance of the groups with which we identify.

In the narrative at the beginning of this chapter, Wendy expressed her view that her doctor took note of her education level when deciding how to speak with her. The fact that Wendy is a highly educated woman appears to be central to her identity, and therefore she had certain expectations of her doctors, and assessed them in terms of their ability to tailor a set of health messages to her based on her group memberships.

SIT has utility for all communication related to illness because of the potential damage illness causes to the identity of individuals who are ill.

Even illnesses such as arthritis or diabetes that may be invisible to the unknowing outsider have the ability to threaten the established identity of people of all ages (Kundrat and Nussbaum, 2003). Recent research on in-patient group identity for mental health patients suggests that the stigmas associated with mental illness affect patients' views of themselves and their place in the community (Jackson et al., 2009). Often, illness disrupts and threatens the order and meaning by which people make sense of their lives (Freund and McGuire, 1999). The overwhelming, uncontrollable, and unpredictable feeling that follows diagnosis of illness frequently paralyzes a person's ability to act and manage their life based on pre-diagnosis norms (Freund and McGuire, 1999; Sparks and Harwood, 2008). Illness can then be a threat to people's ability to plan for the future, and to their sense of control over the activities of daily life.

Responses to illness that affect social identity may impact decisions made by patients and providers. Agency-identity theory suggests that the decision-making processes at the intrapersonal, relational, and cultural levels could all benefit from an agency approach to health communication (Villagran et al., 2007). Since agency in communication translates to an empowered "originator of action, a source of messages" (Stohl and Chency, 2001: 369), acting as an agent or advocate for oneself is useful in every realm of social identity.

Emotions caused by illness, language choices, and perceptions of physical abilities of an ill person are also impacted by a sense of choice in the negotiation of social and personal relationships. In other words, the extent to which our social identity undergoes a shift after a diagnosis, and the nature of our identity shift, is in part a choice we make based on our perceptions of the negative and positive aspects of our condition, as well as the ways in which others orient to our condition through communication. We simultaneously adapt our self-concept to align with our view of the illness, and make choices about how to communicate with others because of our new outlook on life. For instance, a couple facing infertility may feel isolated, stressed, or cheated by their inability to have a child. They may feel left out of their social group of friends if they are the only ones without children. The infertile couple may choose to take on a new identity as the "best babysitters," or they may choose to find a new group of friends who do not have children because of the stigma associated with not having children among their peer group. Decisions about whether to pursue infertility treatments can also have a negative stigma for some people, but the reward of having a child may make that stigma more bearable. Whatever the decision, by communicating with each other and their health-care provider about their concerns, the couple will be more able to play an active role in the impact of infertility on their identities.

Primary, secondary, and tertiary identities

Three levels of identity exist in the health-care context (see, e.g., Harwood and Sparks, 2003; Sparks and Harwood, 2008). At the primary level, individuals identify with large-scale social groups, and those identifications influence their susceptibility and ability to cope with illness. For instance, highly identified *women* might, under some circumstances, be more likely to engage in appropriate prevention strategies for their overall health related to a proper and healthy diet, exercise, or relationships. Women who view their gender as a major part of "who they are" may also be more likely to take part in activities such as the Susan B. Komen Race for the Cure because it is an event that focuses on women's health issues. Highly identified women feel that their gender is one of their most important, defining, characteristics. Women who do not strongly identify with their gender identity are still women, but the details of what it means to engage in the social and cultural roles of women may be less important, or less common.

It is important to note that the biology of being female is quite different from the choice to highly identify as a female. SIT maintains that we choose to align ourselves with certain groups, and choose to minimize characteristics that might make us eligible for other groups because we perceive certain groups to be more desirable. For example, a water polo player may choose to associate more with her teammates and less with her opera and chorus colleagues in an effort to strengthen her identity as an athlete (or vice versa). Females who do not value social and cultural norms of women may choose not to strongly identify themselves as a woman. In this manner, biology is very different from the social construction of identity in our interactions with others.

At the secondary level, identifications with particular behaviors influence health communication processes. Secondary-level identification might mean a patient is less concerned with being recognized as a member of a particular social group, but more likely to feel the need to engage in certain behaviors over time. For example, even if a person does not see himself as a first-rate athlete, he may still feel a strong need to exercise on a regular basis. His identity is shaped more by what he does than who he is as a person. Secondary identity is different from primary identity in that a behavior such as exercise may be central to a person's identity at one phase of life but may become less important as time goes on. Another example of secondary identity is that of "a smoker." Smokers who choose to quit engaging in the behavior typically lose membership with the social group of smokers, so that may mean going from being viewed as socially desirable to being viewed as socially undesirable or vice versa. If smoking is seen as a way to identify with the *cool people*, then stopping the behavior means losing group membership. If, on the other hand, smoking is viewed with a negative stigma, quitting can enable a person to move from the out-group of smokers to the in-group of non-smokers and ex-smokers. Research on the identities of young female smokers suggests that women who are expecting to get pregnant or who have just become pregnant, and who consider themselves to be good mothers, are more likely to quit smoking during pregnancy than young women who did not have this identity (Lennon et al., 2005).

At the tertiary level, identification with health-specific identities becomes important (e.g., patient, victim, survivor, etc.). At this level, the major factor is how a person views his or her social identity as it relates to the symptoms and prognosis of a particular disease. Those who view themselves as fighters will view serious illness differently from the way they would if they viewed themselves as weak or defenseless. At this level, it is less about who we are or what we do, and more about how we choose to frame our behaviors in difficult situations.

Given the nature of patient and provider interactions, the first and third levels of identity are perhaps the most pertinent. Age and socio-cultural identities typically belong in the first level, and more specific health identities, such as cancer, typically belong in the third (Sparks and Harwood, 2008). While previous research on social identity and health dealt largely with the independent effects of different types of identity (Harwood and Sparks, 2003), as well as follow-up elaboration on their interdependence (Sparks and Harwood, 2008), social identity in health-care interactions is also somewhat unique in that it is often invisible and commonly stigmatized. It is clear that identity can play a strong role in effective patient and provider communication.

Stigma and identity

A diagnosis of illness often comes with a negative social stigma (Williams, 2008). Throughout our lives we are exposed to negative information about certain illnesses, so we have preconceived ideas about the stereotypes people face when they are diagnosed with a disease (Harwood and Sparks, 2003). When a person perceives his or her identity is threatened or devalued, based on some change in health status, the natural tendency is to find a way to deal with the threat. A heart disease patient who previously identified as a healthy person (primary identity), ate a healthy diet (secondary identity), and was a tough patient (tertiary identity) experiences shifts in social identity through interaction with others that supports the notion that immortality is not realistic and even healthy people get sick. Identities associated with broader cultural or social collectivist groups are perpetuated by discrimination, stereotyping, and awareness (Harwood and Sparks, 2003). These negative consequences add to the burden of patients who are already dealing with the biological problems associated with their condition, and can cultivate unnecessary stress for patients and their caregivers.

Out-group membership is often related to the stigma attached to the type of illness, and the view of the illness in society. Patients with a sexually transmitted disease, for example, are members of a stigmatized out-group that can negatively impact their social identity. Mental illness can have similar negative stigmas. However, some members of mental illness communities, such as those individuals with Asperger's or mild autism, are proud of their social identities (Wallis, 2009). Certain less visible health issues create a hidden stigma because the patient's social group members cannot see signs of illness, so it may be difficult for them to understand the impact on the patient. Sometimes, health problems that start as very vague cues may be misdiagnosed for months, years, or, in many cases, decades before a proper diagnosis is made. By this time the illness has often had an impact on a patient's interactions, relationships, and overall behaviors. For instance, a friend was diagnosed with celiac disease in later life after decades of problems and issues that were viewed by many doctors as "psychosocial" issues. Although it was a relief to figure out the actual and proper diagnosis, all the years of hearing statements such as "it is in your head," or "you are fine . . . get over it," really had taken a toll on the patient's mental as well as physical health. In this case, *not* belonging to the stigmatized group of ill patients (based on the lack of an accurate diagnosis of illness) can also create a negative self-concept and a high level of uncertainty about confusing symptoms.

Insight and identity

The term *insight* refers to the capacity of a patient to recognize that he or she has an illness in need of treatment (Williams, 2008). Insight involves awareness, acceptance, and willingness to adhere to treatment for illness, and these factors are typically shaped by the perceived stigma associated with a particular disease. Recent research suggests that insight occurs as a cognitive process that is independent of the patient's views of the usefulness of medical treatment (Linden and Godemann, 2007; Williams, 2008) and should be thought of as a transformative development of social identity. Through social interactions, patients see themselves in a different light, and begin to understand that others may view them differently as well. Linking insight to social identity changes a patient's outlook on illness from a purely biomedical perspective to a more holistic experience (Williams, 2008). Insight has mainly been cited in relation to issues of mental health (Williams and Collins, 2002; Mossakowski, 2003); one such study links level of insight with a greater level of perceived stigma felt by mental health patients (Mishra et al., 2009). However, it has informative properties for examining illness and identity in a variety of health-care contexts.

Insights among patients can have differing effects on identity. A typology of post-diagnosis identity for schizophrenics (Williams, 2008) proposed four main types of identity shift that occur based on cognitive and behavioral experiences of patients: engulfed, resistant, empowered, and detached. Although Williams's (2008) research on schizophrenia uses these four identity-shift types to highlight various aspects of insights about illness and social identity, we build on the work of Williams (2008) to propose a typology that includes a more prominent focus on the role of identity in communication with health-care providers. Our contention centers around the notion that patients not only experience illness biologically, cognitively, emotionally, and behaviorally, but they also view illness and its relative importance to their existing identity based on experiences within the clinical setting. The usefulness of medical treatment is not in question, but rather the impact of information sharing in medical encounters is the most important aspect of treatment in terms of social identity. Perceived social stigma is often created and reinforced by the information presented by providers, and by the way illness is explained and framed. For instance, if a provider says "You will feel weak and frail for the next six weeks," and the patient already feels unwell, s/he receives the reinforced message of "weakness" and, as a result, plays out that stigmatized role of "weak patient." Patients who identify as engulfed or empowered will be more likely to actively participate in health-care interactions, while resistant and detached patients are more likely to exhibit poor communication with providers, including a lack of listening, cognitive processing, and active decision-making. Table 7.2 outlines the typology of the role of illness on identity and communication for patients in health care.

Engulfed identities are when the patient identity is prominent, and includes diminished self-esteem and negative stereotypes of self (Williams, 2008). These patients may find comfort inside the health-care system because it creates support and structure from providers, as well as access to social support among other patients. Illness becomes a priority in this patient's life and identity is transformed by the characteristics of disease. In provider–patient interactions, engulfed patients actively seek information, and share in health-care decisions. Providers may view engulfed patients as overly dependent on caregivers or as too eager to surrender all of their pre-diagnosis identity. Doctors may try to encourage engulfed patients to carry on with certain aspects of their pre-diagnosis life to limit negative identity shifts.

Resistant identities also include negative stereotypes of self, but self-esteem is protected by resistance to, or denial of, illness (Williams, 2008). Resistant patients maintain a sense of control over their identity by limiting dialogue about their condition with their providers, and even by deceiving providers about the severity of symptoms. Resistant patients cannot avoid feeling symptoms of illness, but they can limit their communication on the nature and meaning of those symptoms. For these patients, admitting illness means accepting a diminished self-concept, so resistant patients will use communication as a barrier to dealing with illness. This patient will also resist in-group affiliation with other patients who have the same condition, in part due to the perceived validity of negative stereotypes of the disease. Acceptance of group membership as a *sick* person is to accept a stigmatized negative identity. A patient with schizophrenia describes her resistance to her mental illness diagnosis: "I completely recognized that the things I was saying and doing and feeling would be thought to amount to a diagnosis of schizophrenia, but I thought that it was not true – I didn't really have the illness" (Saks, 2009: 972).

Empowered identities are when the patient's illness is taken on with full force and a sense of pride, and negative stereotypes of illness are rejected (Williams, 2008). Empowered patients feel a low internalized stigma, so their communication with others is not framed to combat stigmatized ideals. As a result, empowered patients may be more likely to join social support networks of patients with the same condition, and may be advocates for others as well. Communication with providers is active and generally positive because the illness is reframed in both negative and

Table 7.2 Typology of the role of illness on identity and communication for patients in health care

	Highly stigmatized illness	Less stigmatized illness
High level of interaction with providers	**Engulfed patient identity** • Communication about illness with provider is lengthy, consistent, negative • Negative stereotypes applied to self • More perceived need for social mobility and social competition • Self-esteem diminished by negative perceptions • Patient identity is a primary identity	**Empowered patient identity** • Communication about illness with provider is consistent, active, positive • Negative stereotypes not applied to self • Self-esteem protected by pride • More perceived need for social mobility and social creativity • Patient identity is a primary identity
Low level of interaction with providers	**Resistant patient identity** • Communication about treatment with provider is sporadic, negative, or combative • Negative stereotypes applied to self • Less perceived need for social mobility or social competition • Social creativity framed to resist identity shift • Self-esteem protected by denial, resistance to illness • Patient identity is not a primary identity	**Detached patient identity** • Communication about illness with provider is sporadic, vague, passive • Negative stereotypes not applied to self • Less perceived need for social mobility and social competition • Social creativity framed to avoid acknowledging identity threat • Self-esteem protected by detachment, indifference • Patient identity is not a primary identity

Source: Adapted from Williams (2008)

positive terms. The patient may have lost certain pre-diagnosis views of self, but will have also gained a new community membership among those diagnosed with the same condition.

Detached identities are when the patient rejects or denies illness and maintains his or her previous identity without regard for the reality of the situation (Williams, 2008). This approach not only rejects the characterization of illness, but also rejects any social stigma associated with disease. Detachment comes from low insight into the nature of the illness, and therefore communication with providers is not active or well-informed. Detached patients may not even seek treatment from providers at all because of the need to isolate themselves from reality and maintain their pre-diagnosis identity. Providers may be viewed as a threat to identity maintenance because open discussion of the illness eliminates the possibility of denying social stigma that may come up in the conversation. For this reason, detached patients' communication with providers may be vague, sporadic, or passive.

Coping with negative patient identities

SIT sheds light on the consequences of identity threat for patients. Specifically, SIT suggests that when a person perceives that an identity is devalued or does not provide rewards, three potential coping mechanisms are available (Shinnar, 2008; Villagran and Sparks, 2009). The stress associated with negative patient identities requires the use of these coping strategies to minimize or eliminate association with the undesirable group. The choice among these three coping strategies is grounded in the level of identification an individual has with the group, the degree to which boundaries between the group and other groups are open or closed, and the degree to which the power structure is viewed as legitimate and stable.

Social mobility

In situations of low identification and open boundaries, the path of least resistance is for an individual to leave a stigmatized or unrewarding group (social mobility). This may take the form of actually leaving (e.g., ceasing to pay membership dues in a union; changing nationality; changing from one group to another) or of psychologically "passing" (e.g., closeted gay people; invisible illness). In terms of a patient's identity, actually leaving the undesirable social group of their illness may not be entirely possible until the illness is eliminated, but in general the mobility option can be exercised in two ways. First, there is an obvious desire for a patient to move toward health, and in so doing to leave their patient identity behind. In the long term, regaining full health and getting rid of an illness is a form of social mobility. A residual sense of the patient-based identity is, however, likely in such situations – while the body is well, the identity of how it feels to be sick may remain.

This mobility strategy is obviously differentially available depending on the type and severity of the illness; some illnesses are temporary and some are chronic. Beyond this issue, however, the extent to which this strategy is *perceived* to be available may differ. In particular, older people may perceive this strategy to be more difficult to achieve, and/or those around them may be less likely to view it as an option. Older adults may treat certain symptoms with less concern (e.g., attributing them to "age"), and vigorous treatment options may be denied or downplayed by physicians compared to their treatment of younger people (e.g., due to stereotyping).

Effectively, the boundaries to the "healthy" identity may be less open than they are for younger people.

Certain communication practices may also perpetuate the view that social mobility is not an option for certain groups. Everyday talk may emphasize the limited social mobility options for older adults, or persons with a terminal disease. Physicians may express their reservations about vigorous treatment as an inherent sense of hopelessness or doubt about certain treatments ("You're too old to take it"), or age-graded prognosis estimates ("A 25-year-old might have two years, but I doubt you have that long"). More generally, discourse surrounding the inevitability of decline and illness in old age (Coupland, 2004) may well lead to a less militant approach to fighting the illness. Communicatively, for instance, older people and terminally ill patients may block their own attempts at effective treatment by fatalistic statements ("I've had a good run – at 83 you can't expect much better"). Unfortunately, these discursive strategies block constructive action such as requesting more aggressive treatment, doing research on therapy options, dealing assertively with health providers, and rejecting terminal diagnoses in favor of experimental treatment options.

Failing to disclose diagnosis, concealing side-effects of treatment, and lying about absences from work, and so on, can also be understood as social mobility strategies. Patients concerned about the stigma associated with a diagnosis may pursue numerous strategies to avoid such stigma while they are fighting the disease. Obviously, these activities are unlikely within the immediate social support network, but they may be common in other contexts (e.g., in protecting vulnerable family members from concern, avoiding discrimination at work, etc.).

The social mobility option is not effective for individuals who value their group membership strongly (Villagran and Sparks, 2010; Harwood and Sparks, 2008). When identification is high, mobility is unlikely and one of the other two options (described below) will be adopted. When identity is low, mobility may indeed be the preferred option. Mobility is also unlikely in situations where the boundaries are closed (people simply are unable to leave because other groups will not accept them). This suggests that the permeability of group boundaries might be an influential factor in future theorizing here. When mobility is not an option, individuals will engage in social creativity or social competition.

Social creativity

This coping mechanism involves using cognitive restructuring to reframe the nature of what it means to be ill. Social creativity generally involves one of three strategies (Shinnar, 2008). First, instead of taking any direct action, the patient may alter the perceptions of illness by finding creative ways to make in-group/out-group comparisons (Shinnar, 2008). People may seek out some dimension on which their group *is* valued, despite its generally low status (e.g., "I may have cancer, but at least I am losing weight!"). Second, sometimes patients may redefine their values to allow for a positive assessment of in-group characteristics (a breast cancer survivor may put a bumper sticker on her car that says "cancer free"). The third approach to social creativity is to target alternative out-groups. For instance, there is already a literature illustrating the ways in which people target other, less well-off, in-group members to achieve positive identities. In the case of patients, this might mean that cancer patients feel "lucky" in comparison to patients with more aggressive or visible illnesses such as ALS. Similarly, Coupland et al. (1988) describe the ways in which older people target other older adult groups (e.g., younger old vs older old) as a comparison group – in particular, older adults suffering physical decline will talk about older people with dementia as a salient out-group against whom they compare themselves positively ("At least I can still drive!").

For some patients, people with more negative or extreme prognoses and/or cognitive problems, alcohol or drug problems, and so on, may be a target out-group with which to make favorable comparisons ("I may be an alcoholic, but at least I'm not a drug addict"). In this case, the patient may be choosing to target groups whose illness is perceived to be optional.

As noted above, older adults have already been shown to target other disadvantaged groups in discourse; indeed, they may have a greater range of (real or imagined) "less well-off" out-groups to target, given the age of their peers and the social representations available for their peers' health. For younger people with healthy peers, such positive comparisons may be more difficult to achieve unless peers who exhibit risky behaviors (drugs, unprotected sex, etc.) are used as the referent out-group.

For people who have recovered, the "survivor" identity may well be intrinsically a highly rewarding identity, so there would be no reason to pursue any mobility/creativity strategies. The "survivor" identity has also been shown to correlate with better psychological well-being and post-traumatic illness growth (Park, Zlateva and Blank, 2009). Age may again moderate responses to survivors: a younger survivor may be viewed as a hero, whereas an older survivor may still carry some residual aura of illness and decline – postponed, perhaps, but looming. Such patterns would yield information on whether and how identification with being a survivor displaces or complements other identities, and hence the ways in which identifying with those other groups provides salve to the threat of the mental health identity.

Social competition

In contrast to social creativity, when the power structure is seen as illegitimate or unstable, people will engage in social competition. Social competition is defined as any collective action to change the status quo (Shinnar, 2008). For patients, social competition might mean staging a protest against a health-care policy, or participating in an AIDS awareness march. When a patient's self-concept is threatened by a negative group identity, members of the group may mobilize to bring attention to that characterization.

At the level of social competition, people are publicly seeking a change in the status quo in an effort to gain more status and resources for their group (see Sparks and Harwood, 2008). Campaigns and awareness programs all fall into this area; perhaps the most visible in the cancer context is the pink ribbon campaign. Relative to other group memberships, these campaigns are interesting in that the primary goal is not to achieve more respect or status for people currently in the group, but rather to raise the status of group membership as an issue (primarily to support research that would prevent future people becoming members of the group!).

Similar to prior research on the role of social identity and cancer (Harwood and Sparks, 2003; Sparks and Harwood, 2008), the options for certain patients to campaign for resources are limited. Even requests for basic levels of dignity and equal treatment may be limited by increasing age, low access to health-care facilities, or lack of communication technology used to mobilize like-minded patients. When patients communicate with their providers, they may not have the force of a mobilized patient group behind them, thereby leaving the patient alone to deal with the consequences of his or her patient identity. Social competition may have indirect effects on the patient–provider interaction until the group's efforts lead to large-scale changes in the way illness is depicted and treated in health-care environments.

Case study: mental illness and social identity

A central concept in this chapter is that communication plays a fundamental role in the way we experience health-related identity shifts. A good example of this concept is mental illness. Patients do not usually self-diagnose mental illness as they would if they felt a lump in their breast. It is most often through interactions with others that mental illness becomes apparent to the patient and/or their family and friends. Our communication with others becomes the key to diagnosis of mental health concerns.

Second, unlike AIDS or cancer, mental illnesses cannot be diagnosed entirely with a brain scan or a blood test. Instead, doctors mostly draw on their perceptions of verbal and non-verbal cues to determine to what extent a patient is healthy or sick. We communicate in therapy sessions to explore the nature of mental illness based on lived experiences, and our ability to convey those experiences is essential for a proper diagnosis.

Third, therapeutic approaches to the treatment of mental illness are rooted in continued communication between the patient and a health-care professional. Adherence to medication is also heavily reliant on discussions about the effectiveness of the treatment protocol. Ongoing regulation of medication and therapy are both rooted in communication with others, so our identity hinges on the way we align ourselves with social groups in our discussion of the disease.

Finally, physicians may miss the symptoms of mental illness because of a patient's obvious and perceived group memberships. If a provider thinks a patient acts a certain way because that is how *those people* always act (whoever those people are), the physician might be missing clear cues of illness because they are being misattributed. Negative stereotypes on the part of providers about the patient's social identity become barriers to proper diagnosis and care that can only be overcome through consistent and competent communication.

For all of these reasons, communication is central to the diagnosis and treatment of mental illness because the symptoms are often noticed based on things patients say and do, versus things they feel. Mental health often affects close family, friends, and social support networks long before the patient gets to a doctor's office. The history of interactions that emerge before diagnosis can greatly impact how we view ourselves as well as the way we orient to those around us via communication, which creates our social identities across the life span. The mental health continuum from the most severe cases to the more simplistic has communicative and behavioral characteristics that make it distinctively tied to our social identities. Such stigma creates barriers to open communication about mental illness with family members and other traditional sources of social support, making patient–provider interactions especially important.

Health-care communication ranges from explicit and relatively well-known disease conditions affecting our population such as heart disease and cancer, but also permeates our society in more subtle and less obvious ways via less visible illnesses such as ALS, multiple sclerosis, celiac disease, and mental illness. The asymmetrical nature of communication in health-care contexts requires a coordinated negotiation of social identity for patients and providers. Providers use instrumental talk to give and receive information and maintain their in-group identity status. Patients enter the interaction with an existing social identity that may be transformed by a diagnosis of illness. Shifts in social identity and health can have particular effects on medical decision-making in the doctor–patient relationship. Through communicating with others, patients diagnosed with an illness often see themselves differently and start to recognize that others may view them differently as well. Awareness of potential identity shifts as an individual experiences a change in his or her health status is a coordinated effort involving all interactions within and outside of the health-care environment.

Discussion Questions to Understand Social Identity

An illness diagnosis affects social identity. Upon hearing news of a diagnosis, people will likely notice a shift in their perceptions of themselves and their status in the community. In this situation, it can be helpful to ask oneself some questions, such as those shown below, about the feelings arising from this identity shift.

What about this disease makes me feel different from how I was before my diagnosis?
How will this illness affect my daily physical abilities?

How will this illness affect the ways in which people in the community view me?

Where can I find support from others in dealing with this illness? Are local or online communities available?

How do I view power in this interaction, and how does my conception of power impact the things I say, or do not say?

How can I maintain positive emotional and social self-image and portray this to others while undergoing treatment?

PART IV

MEDIATED AND ORGANIZATIONAL
INFLUENCES ON PATIENT AND PROVIDER
INTERACTION

8 Social Media

Last year when I was 19, I was under a tremendous amount of stress. I was constantly bummed out about school, work, and a tough breakup with my girlfriend of four years. When I didn't have to go to work, I would sleep in all weekend. Sometimes, I would rest on the couch and watch SPIKE TV and ESPN for days, ordering two large pizzas to eat by myself when I was hungry. I must admit, I ate everything I wanted (and then some) and I never had time to go to the gym. In high school I was a lineman on my football team, so I have always been big, but all of a sudden I was not big anymore – I was fat. I was unhealthy, overweight, and stressed out. When I went home at semester break, my mom made me go to the doctor. I was sure my doctor was going to put me on some terrible program of rabbit food and diet pills. When I left the doctor's office I did have a prescription to help me get active and healthy. The surprising thing was what my doctor suggested that I do. He said he understood how stressful college can be and how difficult it is to find time to go to the gym to workout. His solution for me was two things – Dance Dance Revolution (DDR) and Wii Fit. My doctor wanted me to work on my stress and get active in the comfort of my own home using video games. This was the weirdest part – we played both games together in his office so he could show me how they worked. My doctor is actually a good Wii boxer. He told me lots of patients are now using technology like Wii and DDR to help them lose weight and have fun too. Wii Fit even included features that help me track my weight loss and body fat index. I am not the best dancer, but I can work up a sweat in no time on DDR. I have also gotten pretty good at Wii, and my friends come over to play, which helps with my loneliness from losing my girlfriend. I guess I thought that doctors always give patients a prescription for pills, or make them sit on a couch and talk about their problems. I never expected that my doctor would give me really good ideas to help me feel better about myself that did not involve the drug store, only the electronics store.

Narrative from Aaron

The Web and new media open up opportunities for connection as never before in history. Patients can carry on conversations with all types of health providers, blogs, caregivers, and so on, through the Web, Twitter, podcasts from providers, instant messaging, or through social networks. When Marshall McLuhan (1964) wrote the famous words "the medium is the message," it is not likely he was referring to the importance of the role of social media in the provider–patient relationship. McLuhan explained that new media would not just add to the nature of what we do in everyday life, but rather that media would transform the very nature of human communication. The creation of the "global village" made it possible to interact across boundaries to share our lives, our problems, and our experiences. The use of social media and various communication technologies in health care is exploding as members of the global village seek to interact with each other, and these new health technologies and streamlined services are made possible through legislative and technical advances. Professional health groups are looking for innovative ways to expand into this growing domain (Maheu, Whitten and Allen, 2001). Some examples include online support groups (such as caregiver.com and dailystrength.org), or provide forums for people to communicate about their health issues, while e-health and telemedicine allow patients to communicate with doctors online and streamline health record databases. File sharing, health-related email, and spam advertisements for pharmaceutical products may bring a whole new meaning to patients who exclaim, "I think I have a virus!"

As members of the "global village," patients who want to share medical records or screening results with a provider in another city, another state, or another country can easily do so on the Internet. If a patient has questions about a diagnosis or treatment, she might also look at the blog of a patient with a similar condition who lives halfway around the world to find answers to her questions. For instance, a mother who is having trouble breastfeeding and cannot reach her pediatrician might also look for answers in a chatroom. A provider who sees a complex set of symptoms concerning a patient in a rural village in Alaska might decide to engage in a teleconference with providers around the world to discuss the rare situation and share best practices for treatment. Technologies such as Skype and YouTube create new twenty-first-century channels for provider collaboration for diagnosis and treatment of patients around the world. The "global village" of health care means that no patient or provider is ever alone, and the number of available venues for health-care interactions is multiplied. Interactive technology creates opportunities for collaboration, information gathering, and shared decision-making in the provider–patient interaction. However, new e-health technologies also raise questions of medical record confidentiality, since online data storage presents possibilities for hacking and misuse (Maddox, 2002).

Social media advocate Chris Brogan claims that consumer environments are short on trust and that people (patients) are more informed, cynical, and savvy than ever (Brogan and Smith, 2009). Social media availability and use does not, in and of itself, guarantee better communication, however. A new communication tool with a dazzling array of functionalities and opportunities for innovation does nothing to help patients or providers unless it is adopted and used in the course of medical encounters (Lett and Scherger, 2007). Technology is not the panacea or answer to improving health care; however, it is a channel through which improved health care can be achieved. Doctors and patients can opt to use efficient, cost-saving, convenient technology, but the adoption of any innovation is subject to the appraisal of the adopter. In other words, if providers or patients do not see a new communication technology as offering a relative advantage to the status quo, it is not likely the technology will be adopted (Rogers, 1983). Social media can provide more personal connections, more information, and more transparency of the health-care providers and systems, which can greatly impact patient and provider interaction and health outcomes. Brogan and Smith (2009) claim that social media can serve as an effective tool to help bring about change, arguably in the health-care environment. Social media is accessible to anyone who can access a computer, and it is usually free!

This chapter looks at the growth and application of social media and new communication technologies in the medical encounter. We explore the most common technology uses, such as chatrooms and email, while also including more advanced uses of technology to enhance communication between providers and patients. Providers and patients are adopting technological tools that attempt to make health care more effective and secure, and to provide reliable and accessible information when it is needed (Lindquist et al., 2008).

Evolving communication technology in health care

In recent years, the widespread adoption of computers, new software programs, the Internet, PDAs, teleconferencing systems and text messaging has led to a variety of changes in communication within the health-care system. One example is Hello Health, an independently owned health-care clinic in Williamsburg, Virginia, that provides fast and affordable health care for the uninsured. Doctor and patient communications are largely conducted by email and text messages, with follow-ups conducted online. The clinic is also working on developing a Facebook page for doctors and patients to connect, as well as an iPhone application that will allow patients to make appointments at the clinic (Callahan, 2009).

Another innovative example of technology use in the PPI was developed by a physician who implemented Skype videochat software for patients with dementia (Wagner, 2010). In the past, physicians gathered important clues about a patient's health behaviors and environmental challenges through home visits. Providers who have homebound patients, such as those with dementia, may use videochat programs to save patients repeatedly traveling to the hospital for routine visits. Skype, the free computer teleconferencing service, can be installed on laptop computers used by home health workers, and physicians can administer routine follow-up care through Skype when the home health-care worker visits, while family members living far from the patient can be invited to "attend" patient meetings through Skype as well. By using Skype instead of face-to-face communication, providers save the preparation time, waiting-room time, costs of staff and supplies for the visit, as well as the cost and potential danger of transporting a dementia patient to the hospital.

Twitter is a tool for micro-blogging, and it has recently been used in surgery departments for keeping anxious family members informed during lengthy surgical procedures (for example, the Henry Ford Hospital). Twitter messages are 140 characters in length, so they offer a quick and easy way to facilitate routine progress updates to family members. Twitter is also an innovative way to cost-effectively allow more medical students, physicians, and community members to learn about the surgical technology a provider is using. Using Twitter enables staff members to not only give those outside the operating room a view of procedures, but also to take questions from those following the Twitter feed online (Henryford.com, 2010). Twitter has been used to create social support groups where physicians monitor the discussion, and for diabetic patients to monitor their sugar levels (Sugarstats.com, 2010). The technology software may change, but the fact is that interactive technology such as Twitter is here to stay.

Technology shapes the ways in which people obtain health information, and the ways in which they communicate about health in daily life. Communication technologies are likely to continue developing and to significantly impact health-care delivery in the future because the health-care system evolves through advancement, innovation, new protocols, and delivery methods to treat patients. Cost-effective technological advances that foster better communication between patients and providers can improve health-care delivery and lead to improved health outcomes.

Communication technology is cost-effective

It is widely reported that effective uses of communication technology in health care have the potential to greatly curtail skyrocketing health-care costs (Neuhauser and Kreps, 2003). Health organizations hope that the application of these technologies will reduce the costs associated with traditional channels of communication such as the telephone and paper-based patient charts, and will reduce travel costs associated with face-to-face meetings of providers to discuss innovations in care. The costs of the current US health-care system are estimated to be over 1.9 trillion dollars in 2009 (Teslik and Johnson, 2009), and they are projected to rise throughout the decades to come. With the increasing costs of health care, it is essential to find ways to reduce the demands of patients on providers by empowering patients to gain credible information and make informed decisions using computer-mediated sources of health information (Neuhauser and Kreps, 2003).

One very cost-effective and complementary tool for health-care delivery is e-health distributed via the Internet. The term "e-health" refers to, "the use of emerging information and communication technology, especially the internet, to improve or enable health care" (Eng, 2001: 1). At no other time has health information been more accessible to people. Hesse et al. (2005) reported that 63.7 percent of the online users have looked for health information for themselves or others at least once in the previous 12 months. As of 2006, around 113 million Americans, 80 percent of adult Internet users, accessed the Internet for health purposes (Rains, 2008).

Despite newly available communication channels, physicians are still the most highly trusted information source for patients (Pecchioni and Sparks, 2007), with 62.4 percent of adults expressing a high level of trust in their physicians (Hesse et al., 2005). For this reason, the Internet does not usually replace physicians as the source of diagnosis or treatment, but patients and their family members can prepare for a visit to the doctor, or follow up on information received from a doctor, through the Internet (Pecchioni and Sparks, 2007). Some providers suggest that the Internet is a good reference source for patients who want more information about their health concerns. For example, recently an older adult patient received a diagnosis for an eye condition from a young ophthalmologist. As the doctor was leaving the examination room, the patient asked, "What was the name of my problem again? It is such a long word I don't think I will remember it." The doctor replied, "Here – I will write down the name and you can Google it when you get home." In this case, the patient had no idea what "Google it" meant, but millions of Americans "Google" health issues every day. In fact, in 2008, Google pledged to help track the spread of flu outbreaks based on users' search patterns for flu symptoms. Their contention was that, as the flu becomes more prevalent in a particular area of the country, more people search for information about flu symptoms. By tracking the number of users entering flu symptoms as search terms, Google can assist public health officials in tracking the spread of the disease (<http://www.google. org/flutrends/>).

Patients who choose to Google health information have access to much of the same knowledge available to physicians through government and research institution websites or from electronic databases available on the Internet. However, many consumers limit their search for health information by using search engines to find health-related websites such as WebMD or KidsHealth (Fox and Rainie, 2000).

Due to increasing Internet access to health information, patients are becoming quite knowledgeable in terms of their ability to discuss specific details of diseases and conditions (Napoli, 2001). Aspden and Katz (2001) have found that such access to health information through the Internet has resulted in creating more informed discussions during physician office visits and medical interviews (see also Ferguson, 1998). In reality, consumers can find a variety of accessible and highly reliable information on government websites, such as the National Institutes of Health (NIH) and the Centers for Disease Control (CDC). However, it is important to be aware that some online sources are less reliable, or totally unreliable, sources of information as well, and it is sometimes difficult to know the difference. The safest method is to check NIH and CDC websites for the most credible and up-to-date information, then to use the more commercial websites to supplement and possibly interpret the credible health information provided by government and academic journals. Other reliable sources include NGO sites such as the Alzheimer's Association, American Cancer Society, and American Diabetes Association.

Opportunities for Internet innovation

Although the Internet is frequently used as a supplementary source of treatment information for patients and doctors, there are still many opportunities for innovative uses of the Internet in patient care. For example, patient-centered information about economic costs of treatment and work-loss for patients remains underdeveloped (Bradley, 2005) – imagine if uninsured patients could look up the average out-of-pocket cost for treating common problems. A website could list average prices in a specific geographic region for casting a broken arm, or getting a mammogram. Some websites do list prices of elective procedures such as plastic surgery, but the full treatment costs associated with non-elective procedures and serious illnesses are more difficult to find (Bradley, 2005). The New Hampshire government has developed such a website, where consumers can research average health-care costs in the state, depending on whether or not they are insured (New Hampshire Health Information Center, 2009). A more transparent system would increase knowledge and potentially bring health-care costs down to more manageable levels for consumers.

Lack of knowledge about treatment costs can add enormous strain to provider–patient communication, and impacts patient choices and decisions regarding whether to visit a doctor in the first place. Doctors cannot treat patients who do not visit their office, but patients without insurance often choose not to be seen precisely because of the lack of transparency about costs. Internet delivery of information could add transparency to health-care costs, while at the same time protecting providers from the need to supply cost-breakdown estimates for every health-care procedure performed for a patient. Communication technology can also be used to link patients in need with sources of financial assistance from private, public, and non-profit sources (Bradley, 2005).

The extent to which all patients feel comfortable with the Internet as a medium for provider communication is also an important area of concern. Internet self-efficacy is increasing rapidly. In 2000, only 25 percent of Americans looked for health information online, but, in 2009, 61 percent of patients went online to research health (Pew Research, 2009). Internet self-efficacy is a person's self-perceived ability to use the Internet for health information (Rains, 2008). Similarly, optimization is described as combining one's skills and resources within a limited goal or life domain to remain effective (Levine et al., 2009). Internet users who perceive they have achieved optimal computer skills may be more likely to feel a greater sense of Internet self-efficacy, which plays a major role in the ways patients and caregivers use online sources of information. Patients with an increased desire for informational involvement tend to have higher self-efficacy, and, in turn, greater perceived success, and more positive attitudes toward the quality of information on the Internet (Rains, 2008). The connection between the desire for information and self-efficacy is important because the Internet is useful for those who wish to take an active role in creating and maintaining positive relationships with providers.

Research suggests that patients requiring more medical information than is typically provided by doctors tend to use the Internet to get that information (Levine et al., 2009). Although patients who desire more written descriptions about their prognosis or treatment can find supplementary information on Internet sites, the credibility of information on the Internet can be questionable and inaccurate information can cause problems when it contradicts information provided by a doctor in a medical encounter.

Although research has indicated that much of the health information on the Internet is either inaccurate or incomplete (Bierman, Golladay and Baker, 1999; Hersch, Gorman and Sacherek, 1998), in recent years there has been an increase in the number of credible sources for health information. Websites affiliated with trustworthy research institutions, medical research firms, and government agencies are often seen as more credible than those who do not have an affiliation with them. The credibility of health information on the Web can be difficult to understand as it is often complex and confusing. It is relatively easy for anyone to post anything on the Internet (and to seem as if they know what they are talking about – in other words, sound credible!). Researchers have credibility concerns regarding consumers' ability to properly evaluate health information on the Internet (Barnes et al., 2003; Cummins et al., 2003). The key is to assess all such information critically, and to remain wary of the content on homegrown websites, when searching for health information.

Despite its potential limitations, the Internet is a key communication channel that influences and complements medical encounters. Patients are no longer passive receivers of information found on the Internet, but rather they create and co-create meaning about illness by asking questions, sharing stories, and choosing whether to engage in online discussions about various health issues. A message from an expert about the need to engage in a particular behavior, or the risk of engaging in another behavior, does not, in and of itself, create a substitute, however, for visits to the doctor. Patients use health information in unique ways, such as gathering preliminary research to take to a doctor visit, or as a sort of "fact check" of information supplied by a provider, when a patient may go online to chat about their diagnosis and treatment (Pecchioni and Sparks, 2007). Patients who use interactive technology to supplement the providers' advice are not passive, but rather active, information seekers who collect information from multiple channels and sources to use when making health-care decisions (Pecchioni and Sparks, 2007).

One study, for example, employed an interactive website designed to be used by asthma patients before a physician visit, so they could prepare relevant questions (Hartmann et al., 2007). It was hoped that preparing patients to ask the right questions would increase their likelihood of receiving tests and treatments suggested by evidence-based guidelines. The study found that patients who went to their visit prepared with information from the website felt more positively about their medical encounters, in part because the website prompted patients to become more actively involved in their discussion with their provider (Hartmann et al., 2007).

Communication technology channels

Although email travels on the Internet between providers and patients, it is a unique channel of communication that is distinctly different from websites. Email is a relatively simple computer application, but it has transformed communication among providers and it is becoming more prevalent among patients and providers. More and more providers are communicating in this way with existing patients to obtain information quickly, check on the patient's progress, or confirm upcoming appointments (Kuzsler, 2000). Once the provider has seen a patient in the clinic several times, he or she can be confident about the patient's ability to use and respond to questions about symptoms, using email (Kuzsler, 2000). Providers in a study of "email savvy" providers reported using email with patients daily to more easily reach patients and avoid "telephone tag," and to help patients manage chronic diseases (Patt et al., 2003). In addition, the asynchronous nature of email might allow apprehensive patients with more time to compose their thoughts when expressing concerns or asking questions about their health (Wright, Sparks, and O'Hair, 2008). Email communications and video conferences between patients and providers about non-emergency health issues add to the ever-expanding "medical home" model, where patients can receive medical information and follow-up consultations in the comfort of their homes (Leviss, 2009).

Many physicians continue to resist utilization of email in their practices. A 2006 study of email use among physicians in an ambulatory unit found that while 63 percent of the physicians who responded used email from their office for communication with friends, family, and other doctors, only 16.6 percent reported communicating with patients using email (Brooks and Menachemi, 2006). Some providers have expressed concerns about the confidentiality of patient information sent through email, as well as the amount of time required and the associated billing issues (Patt et al., 2003). Moreover, email lacks the personal connectedness of a face-to-face visit, which has the potential to affect the accuracy of care recommendations and can lead to malpractice suits if patients are misdiagnosed electronically (Leviss, 2009).

Personal digital assistants (PDAs)

Although widely used by medical and nursing students, greater use among all providers of the personal digital assistant (PDA) has tremendous potential to enhance information access for medical encounters (Lindquist et al., 2008). PDAs are a fairly affordable and convenient tool for providers to retrieve medical information on the spot. When talking with patients, providers using PDAs have access to the latest medical information, including treatment options, drug protocols, and potential side-effects of specific drug interactions (Lindquist, 2008). Providers need a variety of types of information throughout the day, and PDAs offer a convenient way to gather and access this information. Research indicates as many as 85 percent of providers who were frequent PDA users said PDA use had influenced their overall clinical decision-making, and 73 percent mentioned access to information from a PDA as a factor in a change to a patient's treatment plans (Dee, Teolis, and Todd, 2005). Moreover, nursing students who were PDA users had more pharmacological knowledge during clinical practice than nursing students who did not use the device (Farrell and Rose, 2008). Evidence suggests that the use of PDAs in health-care settings can improve patient-centered interactions and decision-making, and reduce the numbers of medical errors caused from inaccurate information in critical situations (Lindquist et al., 2008). More and more providers are utilizing such devices for text messaging or SMS, for short silent message delivery within hospitals and other health organizations. Texting is becoming increasingly popular among users of all levels, from early to late adopters (also known as laggards) of new technologies, with differing age ranges, ethnic backgounds, and so on. In fact, text message technology has even been adopted by an understaffed clinic in Malawi, Africa, to maximize providers' ability to respond to patients and distribute prescription information to pharmacies (Johnson, 2009).

Prescriptions for patients can be easily emailed to hospital pharmacies, and the process of making additional appointments and referrals is facilitated through wireless technology, enabling messages to be sent quickly and conveniently to receptionists and other medical staff. In the past, physicians often made notes in charts after a meeting with patients, and then used transcription services to provide detailed information about patients. Wireless devices help providers to supply more detail about medical conditions for patient records, and they also help to circumvent illegibility of poor handwriting, or other problems associated with taking notes about patients.

Electronic records

For decades, a patient's paper-based medical chart has been the standard site for patient record-keeping. Situation comedies or TV shows such as *Curb Your Enthusiasm* and/or *Seinfeld* have even focused on the doctor's peculiar medical chart notes about a patient's habits or distinct personality traits or interests. Indeed, it is normal to wonder what is written in one's own chart, especially because it appears that doctors go out of their way to prevent patients seeing the document during the medical encounter. Electronic patient medical records are replacing the old handwritten records as a way to locate all information about a patient in an easily accessible virtual space. Electronic records indeed have tremendous potential in terms of standardizing, collating, and storing patient health information.

Although there are some new and innovative uses for computer technology in the PPI, recent data on the cost-effectiveness of perhaps the most popular technological innovation, electronic medical records, are inconclusive at best (Himmelstein, Wright, and Woolhandler, 2009). Electronic medical records have been promoted as a tool to save health-care costs and improve quality of care, but there is little evidence they also improve the PPI. Specifically, when a provider is staring at a computer screen, he or she is not interacting with the patient. All of the non-verbal cues and immediacy that should occur in the interaction are lost when the provider never even looks at the patient. A skillful provider can make the shift between the desktop computer and the patient, but this skill is not currently being taught in medical schools or nursing schools. One potential solution is the use of computer tablets that providers put in their laps while speaking with patients. This increases the possibility of interaction and eye contact with patients if the provider knows how to use the tablet.

Although a majority of patients like the idea of having access to their own medical records via the Internet, there are some patients who have concerns regarding the confidentiality of their information. Patient fears are not completely unfounded. For instance, pre-existing health conditions can impact patient options for health insurance. The Department of Health and Human Services (DHHS) has been collaborating in recent years with various federal agencies as well as private industry to identify necessary, efficient, and acceptable standards for health information to be shared safely and securely among health-care providers.

Although patient preferences for electronic records are indeed varied, personally controlled health records (PCHR) allow patients who use technology to maintain and manage their own records and medical histories, and PCHR can also provide a virtual space to communicate with providers about important health issues (Rodriguez, Casper, and Brennan, 2007).

Patients can choose providers to whom access to PCHR is given, and, based on the information in the records, the provider is able to send per-sonalized prevention and treatment recommendations to the patient's inbox that cue the patient about when to come for a visit (Bourgeois et al., 2008). A study of uses of PCHR for flu shot reminders allowed doctors to post a note in the patient's inbox with a reminder to get a flu shot, send a personalized risk assessment based on the current flu strain, or provide a flu map to give up-to-date information about flu outbreaks in the area (Bourgeois et al., 2008). Reminders for prescription refills, screening tests, and potential health risks can be sent to the patient via a number of avail-able technologies, ranging from voicemail to email to text messaging or SMS.

Interestingly, the primary predictors of whether a patient will support the idea of Internet-accessible records are not the person's age, race, or education level (Ross et al., 2005). Instead, a patient's previous experience with the Internet and their views of the potential benefits and drawbacks of online access to information seem to be the best indicators of whether a patient would favor Internet access to medical records. Electronic records are definitely the wave of the future, so new systems for confidentiality and patient privacy are being created every day.

Web therapy

Web-based self-help therapy for persons with mental health issues is becoming a popular alternative to more traditional channels of self-help information (van Straten, Cuijpers, and Smits, 2008). A recent study of patients with symptoms of depression, anxiety, and work-related stress found web-based self-help therapy to be effective at decreasing depression and anxiety, but results about its effect on stress were inconclusive (van Straten et al., 2008). There is some evidence that the text-based nature of computer-mediated communication has advantages for patient and providers in these types of interventions. Weinberg et al. (1995) argued that the therapeutic value of writing down problems in text-based computer-mediated support groups may derive from its allowance of more distance from others, enabling reflection without concern for the immediate responses of others.

In another study of web-based self-help therapy, it was noted that the Internet improves on more traditional self-help books and CDs because it allows for more interactive approaches to therapy that include sound and video clips (Clarke et al., 2002). Indeed, more recent versions of online therapy even use interactive technology, such as the use of avatars and MMO Virtual Massively Multiplayer Online Virtual Sex Games (MMOVSG) in therapeutic settings (Suler, 2004). A MMOVSG simulation can be used to create virtual sexual intercourse between Player characters. In mental health settings, therapists can use interactive technology to reduce the inhibition of patients with sexual dysfunction to help get to the root of health problems. The disinhibition effect states that people say and do things in virtual settings that they might not be comfortable saying or doing in face-to-face interactions (Suler, 2004). Further, health-care professionals can use communication technology to help patients tap into mental health issues such as those sometimes associated with sexual problems. Communication technologies cross borders and cultures. For example, the Rutger Nisso Group, in the Netherlands, started in 2007 with digital therapy for young victims of sexual harassment (<http://www.rutgersnissogroep.nl/English>). In France, le Centre d'etudes et de recherché pour intensification du traitement du diabete (Center of Studies and Research for Diabetes Treatment) tried out a mobile that improves the monitoring of diabetic patients and that gives the patient more autonomy (<http://www.voluntis.com/Portals/0/documents/diabeo%20english.pdf>). Through technology, patients are likely to be more uninhibited and to express themselves more openly (Suler, 2004), which in turn may improve health outcomes.

Telemedicine

During the past decade telemedicine has become an important means for health-care interactions, and various types of telemedicine are projected to increase dramatically over the next 10 years (Turner, 2003). Technological advances such as telemedicine help cut costs associated with traditional care by providing new channels of communication between patients and providers, and among providers in different geographic regions. For example, telemedicine has become an important cost-saving measure in countries around the world for increasing access to specialists while reducing travel costs for patients and providers. This approach to medical encounters is usually achieved through the use of videoconferencing and Web cameras, in combination with email to send and receive important test results and documents. A recent news article recounted the story of an 80-year-old Alzheimer's patient from Marsala, Sicily, who was able to avoid a 500-mile trip to a specialist by using telemedicine (Crane, 2005). The woman's care was delivered through a television camera at a nearby clinic that was connected to Italy's top Alzheimer's treatment center. Telemedicine allowed this woman's local doctor to benefit from the expertise offered by a health specialist or technician located on the other side of her country. The providers used this technology to cheaply and conveniently conduct her examinations, and to obtain patient data such as reports from laboratories, pharmacies, and technicians at any location. This is only one example of how telemedicine has the potential to offer more comfortable and affordable options for patients in remote areas to be seen by top experts in health care who can read electrocardiograms, blood-pressure levels, and X-rays, and talk directly with patients in real time. Worldwide, governments and technology companies are investing heavily in telemedicine because of its cost-saving potential for a growing elderly population (Crane, 2005). For instance, in the Netherlands, patients are familiar with "the telenurse". The patient, at home, is connected by his videocam with a nurse. He can speak with her and see her on his TV screen. The patient can show her his medication if he has some doubts and she can give him "live" advice (<http://www.zorgkrant.nl/read.html?id=7097>).

New channels for message tailoring

Advances in communication technology channels, such as text messaging, allow providers to tailor messages to specific characteristics of their patient, and then deliver the message in a familiar and accessible format. Diverse audiences need to be reached in new ways, sometimes through music, song, or even humor (H. Osbourne, personal communication, November 16, 2009). According to Kreuter et al. (2000), tailored health promotion material refers to "any combination of information and behavior change strategies intended to reach one specific person, based on characteristics that are unique to that person, related to the outcome of interest, and derived from an individual assessment" (p. 5). Rimal and Adkins (2003) contend that it is important to understand various aspects of the target audience, the channel(s) that will be used in the campaign, and the individual messages that participants will receive. These authors define segmentation as "dividing members of the target according to some meaningful criterion," targeting as "selecting the proper channel, based upon audience characteristics," and tailoring as "crafting health messages to reflect audience characteristics" (p. 500). Tailored communication messages must be designed and delivered to match the specific communication skills, needs, and predispositions of the target population.

Formal and informal providers who are utilizing technologies to bring about health behavior change must take into consideration the specific design of messages and interventions that will encourage patients to be active participants in the medical communication encounter (Sparks and Turner, 2008). The goal of tailored messaging in this context must also be pursued by focusing on an understanding of the unique cognitive and emotional processes of a given target population, followed by particular message framing that is likely to reach the population. It is imperative to understand that certain target populations such as older adults have unique barriers that mandate careful thought prior to message design. We must create messages that can be seen, recalled, and systematically processed (see, e.g., Sparks and Turner, 2008).

A recent example of providers using specifically tailored messages to reach their patients via new technology is the Sweet Talk system, which delivers tailored motivational messages from providers to young people with Type 1 Diabetes, using text messaging (Franklin et al., 2008). Since young people are common users of text-messaging systems, this program offers providers the opportunity to communicate with a younger format that is more convenient and familiar than face-to-face meetings or telephone calls. Sweet Talk users received automated, scheduled text messages from providers offering support, information, and reminders about medical adherence (Franklin et al., 2008). Patients' use of the system for submission of clinical data and to ask important questions demonstrated that Sweet Talk became a trusted medium for younger diabetes patients and their providers.

Social networks

Social media is defined by Joseph Thornley, an online media expert, as "online communications in which individuals shift fluidly and flexibly between the role of audience and author. To do this, they use social software that enables anyone to post, comment on, share or mash up content and to form communities around shared interests" (2008). Brian Solis, a pioneer of new media, adds that new media is a "perpetually evolving mechanism that advances the sharing of information online" (2007). When used strategically, new media, including blogs, social networks, and podcasts, have the potential to increase the value of health organizations by providing useful and relevant health information to interested parties – patients, providers, the media, and so on – and to engage them in the health conversation (Brogan, 2008). Humans are social animals, largely influenced by members of their social groups; therefore, social networks have the power to influence health trends, such as weight loss and tobacco consumption. If my cousin or friend adopts a healthier diet and exercise plan, I am more likely to do the same and encourage others to do so as well (Christakis and Fowler, 2009).

Social networking sites, including Facebook, Twitter, and YouTube, are increasingly being used by patients, providers, and health organizations to communicate about health. Facebook is a free, online social networking site that allows users to create profiles and connect with friends and organizations by commenting on their profiles, uploading photographs, and reading updates posted by the site users. The Ohio State University Medical Center, for example, uses two Facebook pages to keep fans up to date on hospital news and events. These pages were especially useful for keeping people informed about the availability of H1N1 vaccinations, especially since their largest online demographic – college students – represented one of the most at-risk groups for contracting H1N1 (Ragan, 2010).

Twitter is another social networking site that allows users to "tweet" 140-character updates, providing an ever-changing news feed where users can search and "follow" topics ranging from H1N1 to cancer. Health organizations such as the American Cancer Society, the National Cancer Institute, and the American Heart Association use Twitter to update their "followers" on current health news and trends. Hospitals and providers are expanding their use of social media as well (Pho, 2009). However, Twitter also has negative implications for some providers. Some patients are using Twitter to complain about negative experiences with certain providers and are listing providers and their offices by name. Moreover, new search functions in Google include Twitter posts, so if a patient were to Google the name of a doctor, they could discover these negative comments in their search (Pollard, 2009). Since 24 percent of e-patients, defined as those patients who have an Internet connection, have consulted online rankings and reviews of providers (Pew Research, 2009), and there are over two dozen websites solely dedicated to provider reviews, providers will increasingly need to pay attention to reputation management (Pollard, 2009).

YouTube provides a forum for users to search for and post videos online for free, and health organizations are using it as a medium to communicate with their consumers. Johnson & Johnson, for example, created the JNJHealth Network, and has posted some 240 videos on topics ranging from depression to diabetes, with over 1,300,000 viewers (Senak, 2009). The CIGNATV health network on YouTube created social relevance during the H1N1 epidemic through its DocRock video, where a doctor raps to give children tips for preventing H1N1. Combined with hospital websites and blog posts from care providers, social networks are an important and expanding medium for health communications (Leman, 2009).

Conclusion

New communication technologies are likely to continue influencing how consumers seek health information and communicate with other consumers and providers about health issues. In addition, these technologies appear to offer health organizations and providers many advantages in terms of gathering, storing, and disseminating health information, such as electronic patient charts and information from diagnostic tests. In addition, telemedicine presents new opportunities for providers to collaborate during the process of caring for patients, and the Internet and other new computer technologies will continue to be used for public health campaigns. However, despite the optimism over these technologies for improving health care, many cultural, educational, financial, and legal barriers exist that will certainly shape the future of new technologies and health communication.

Discussion Questions for Finding Credible Health Information Online

The Internet is a powerful tool for empowering patients to seek information about their health conditions and health needs. However, not all information is accurate, so it is important for patients to recognize which sources are valid and which are not. The following questions can be used when conducting online health information searches by assessing the reliability of website content to help ensure you are getting the facts.

What is the source of the information? Is this a credible source?

What do my instincts tell me about this information? Does it seem true or believable?

Is the information backed by a well-respected health website such as the Center for Disease Control?

Is there a second or third reference that can confirm the same information?

Is the information a fact or an opinion?

If the information includes a testimonial, how credible does the source of the testimonial appear? Are they sincere?

How current is the information? When was it last updated?

What further questions do I have that I need to address with my doctor?

What are the implications for my privacy of using this technology?

9 Health-care Organizations and Teams

Two doctors and a health insurance administrator died and lined up at the pearly gates for admission to Heaven. St Peter asked them to identify themselves. One doctor stepped forward and said, "I was a pediatric spine surgeon and helped kids overcome their deformities." St Peter said, "You can enter." The second doctor said, "I was a psychiatrist. I helped people manage their depression and other mental illnesses." St Peter also invited him in. The third applicant stepped forward and said, "I was the director of a large health insurance company. I tried to make sure people got cost-saving health care." St Peter said, "You can come in too." But, as the insurance company director walked by, St Peter added, "You can only stay three days. After that you can go straight to Hell!"

Anonymous

President Barack Obama claimed, upon introducing the Obama-Biden Health Reform Bill in 2009, that the plan would provide affordable, accessible health care for all Americans, and build on the existing health-care system, while utilizing existing providers, doctors, and health organizations to implement the plan. The Obama plan embedded promises leading to reduced health-care costs by $2,500 for a typical family, and encouraged investments in health information technology, prevention, and care coordination, while also promoting public health by requiring coverage of preventative services, including cancer screenings, as well as increasing state and local preparedness for terrorist attacks and natural disasters (<http://www.barackobama.com/issues/healthcare/>). In considering approval of the plan, Democrats and Republicans debated in terms of appropriate coverage for all, reduction of rising costs, comparisons of global health-care systems, level of government involvement, impact of malpractice, making insurance work for the people, issues of pre-existing conditions, HIPPA, and health-care reform. Although the specifics of federal involvement in health care change from year to year, and from nation to nation, each of these topics has direct implications for the provider and patient interaction. Although most would agree that health care is a fundamental part of society, a wide variety of problems exist in terms of our ability to provide adequate health care for everyone who needs it. The rising cost of health care will continue to have a substantial impact on almost all patients in the coming years as health-care organizations try to find innovative ways to reduce the cost of their services. Since the medical encounter occurs within a larger organizational structure, it is important to examine how health organizations shape our communication with providers.

Imagine an organization where there are several bosses, several different sets of rules, a variety of costs for the same item, and multiple procedures for the same task. Patients can get frustrated by the complexity of their own care, and providers need to be up to date on ever-changing regulations, reimbursement procedures, and contractual obligations to health delivery systems, pharmaceuticals, and health-care teams. A patient's provider is the point of entry into the complex web of health care. The interactions among the health-care team also occur as part of that web. For example, a recent story of a woman who was in labor highlights the interrelationship between providers and their health delivery system. The woman was only six and a half months' pregnant and she thought she was having labor pains. She called her doctor and he advised her to go directly to her local hospital. The local hospital was very small, and was not equipped with a neonatal intensive care unit. When the woman arrived at the hospital, the clerk asked the reason for her visit. The woman was in a great deal of pain by this time and she replied, "I am only 30 weeks pregnant and I think I am in labor. My doctor told me to come in to get medical attention as soon as possible." The clerk responded to the woman by saying, "Well, I don't know why your doctor told you to come here. I cannot admit you because you cannot have that baby here. You need to go to a hospital that is equipped to take care of premature babies." The woman was stunned because she knew that the nearest hospital with this type of facility was over two hours' drive away. She left the hospital and ended up delivering her baby in the car. The rules and structure of the organization created a barrier to health care for the woman and her child. The clerk was subsequently fired, and the baby was fine.

The Joint Commission on the Accreditation of Healthcare Organizations (JCAHO) (2002) indicates that 80 percent of medical errors are due to communication breakdown. Miscommunication in health-care organizations is serious business, resulting in millions of lost revenues, lost loved ones, lost limbs, and huge numbers of malpractice lawsuits, with malpractice litigation averaging an annual cost of $30.4 billion (Towers Perrin, 2008). Medical malpractice lawsuits can also impact insurance rates because doctors are required to carry expensive malpractice insurance policies to protect themselves if they are sued (Larsen, 2009). These expenses are then passed on to patients; an average 10 percent of a doctor's bill goes to cover the cost of medical malpractice insurance (Furchtgott-Roth, 2009). To study the provider–patient interaction in the context within which it occurs means taking a look at the structures and functions of health-care organizations. Patient participation in health-care organizations requires a sense of agency on the part of the patient (Stohl and Cheney, 2001). Participation is based on both the cognition of the patient (his or her own thoughts about how the medical encounter should go) and the structure of health care within the organization (ibid.). The woman in the previous story was confronted with a situation where she needed to be an advocate for her own health concerns. Her participation in the health-care organization was hindered by the clerk who seems to have been more concerned about the legal or procedural aspects of the situation than she was about the care of the patient. The woman was probably not at her strongest, most self-confident moment as she was going into labor in the waiting room, and the system was not set up to help her overcome that obstacle.

Sometimes patients are in a position to advocate for themselves, and sometimes they are not. For example, patients and family members dealing with long-term illnesses are in a different health-care situation from others dealing with the often complex and confusing health-care environment. Through the empowerment of relational resources, patients and their partners elevate their prospects for exerting agency in the conduct of their interactions with each other and with the health-care system. Agency refers to choice, being in a position where multiple options and alternatives have been created through strategic communication. Partners and family members may begin to feel that their perceptions of, and behaviors with, each other are working well, and therefore they can focus on emotional closeness and on strategizing how they will manage long-term illnesses. For instance, a family member may insist on second opinions when they are faced with a disappointing prognosis report, or they may appeal against insurance restrictions on participating in a clinic trial. Communication efforts such as these represent the ability to expand choices.

Agency also entails having the capability and resources necessary for making competent decisions based on a wider range of choices. Patients differ in their willingness and ability to be active participants in the health-care process (Brashers, Hass and Neidig, 1999). The diagnosis, prognosis, and treatment of such long-term illnesses are often difficult to predict. The burdens of making decisions that promote the health of the patient, while at the same time accommodating the relationship among all involved in the decision-making, is an overwhelming task. Agency reflects the confidence that patients and their family members have in their decision-making skills and empowers patients to seek the best approach for care (Kidney Cancer Association, 2009).

Finally, agency represents enhanced opportunities for influencing the context that family members manage to construct through their communication. Influence is the persuasive management of the choices involved in such decision-making processes. Patients and caregivers forge ahead with plans and strategies for managing the illness in ways that are conducive with their needs and desires, rather than succumbing to the limitations in an often confusing, inflexible, and complex health-care system. Agency places partners in a position where they assume control of their care plan, their personal lives and, importantly, their relationships. To further complicate such issues, sometimes there is a *double-bind* that may impact patient participation because the patient simultaneously desires to be part of the decision-making processes about his or her health, but may also want clear answers from providers about what to do next. Patients and providers negotiate participation in health organizations based on this paradox.

At first, patients may not feel completely empowered as a partner in their own health organization. Enrollment paperwork, choosing a

Table 9.1 Framework for patient agency in health-care organizations

Entry	Uncertainty	Empowerment	Agency
Shock	Problematic integration	Decision-making	Self-advocacy
Powerlessness	Uncertainty	Advocacy	Control
Stigma	management	Voice	Influence
Fear	Assimilation	Adaptation	Competence
	Coping		

Source: O'Hair et al. (2005)

provider, being assigned a provider, co-pays, and disallowed procedures can be confusing and complex. Over time, however, uncertainty can turn to empowerment as more information is acquired (Villagran and Hoffman, 2009), and then to agency based on the nature of the provider–patient relationship. Patients can move from a sense of fear and shock following a serious diagnosis to adapt and gain a more controlled self-perception of advocate, or agency, for successful treatment. Organizational communication scholars describe *agency* as a state of actualization that empowers the individual to have choice and, if desired, exert control over the health environment. Stohl and Cheney (2001: 369) note that:

> Agency entails a sense of being, efficacy, and the feeling that an individual can or does make a difference (Giddens, 1984). Agency captures the notion of the self as originator of action, a source of messages, a force to be reckoned with. In dialectical tension with structure, agency is one of the central concepts of social theory; its implications for communication are important in that they implicate the ideas of free will and one's capacity to make a difference within a social setting (Whalen and Cheney, 1991).

Based on differences in family structure, education, upbringing, and world-view, patients grow from childhood to adulthood with vastly different perceptions of the extent to which they can play a role in their own health care (Barr, 2008). Those patients who have been raised to believe they are in charge of their own lives are more likely to believe they have viable alternatives and voice, or agency, in medical encounters (Villagran, Fox, and O'Hair, 2007). A sense of agency, then, opens the door of opportunity for choice within the patient–health-care context. In order to arrive at a place where agency can be maximized, patients need to see themselves as capable partners in their own care, then consider the extent to which it is most beneficial to lead or follow in various aspects of their care (Villagran et al., 2007).

Sometimes patients may choose to lead a discussion about a specific medicine that has uncomfortable side-effects. Usually, the patient will choose to follow the expert advice of a provider. In either case, agency is enacted through communication with others. Acting as a co-equal team member means becoming an active participant in the health-care process by speaking and listening to all members of the health-care team.

Many physicians have their own office and office staff with a particular set of rules and a chain of command. The doctor will refer patients to a hospital that has its own organizational structure, of which the doctor and patient are a part. Each of the three parties – the hospital, the doctor's office, and the doctor – will communicate directly with the other two, and each will need to relay information to the third party that they get from the second party. Sounds confusing? It can be confusing for anyone, and patients are not always aware why their provider cannot answer a specific question, or find a test result. Poor communication among organizational members directly impacts a provider's ability to offer patients maximum information about test results, with minimum delay. Patients who feel a sense of agency are more capable of maneuvering within the health-care structure.

An example of this is Enrique, an educated man in his late thirties. Enrique's job as a hardware store manager requires some physical labor, but for several months he had trouble with his shoulder when lifting anything heavy in his store. Enrique realized that over time his shoulder could potentially become even more painful, and could ultimately keep him from being able to do his job, so he went to the doctor to get it checked out. He told the doctor that he had shoulder pain, and the doctor told him he needed an MRI, which would be conducted at a lab across town. Enrique felt he had taken charge of the situation and was on his way to getting it resolved. He left work early and drove across town to have the test. The technician who would conduct the test asked Enrique to point to the spot where he was feeling pain. He pointed to the side of his chest, near the top of his arm. The technician then told Enrique, "Well, you are actually pointing to the top of your pectoral muscle, not your shoulder. The doctor requested an MRI of your shoulder and we cannot MRI the spot you are pointing to now." Enrique explained that he and the doctor had talked about the "shoulder" in broad terms, but the technician was adamant that he could not do an MRI of that spot without an order from the doctor. The technician did the MRI, but since the area where Enrique was in pain was not included in the scan everything looked fine. Many patients would just give up at this point, but Enrique went back to his doctor, got another MRI ordered for the pectoral region, and began the whole process again. Each MRI cost almost $1,000, so Enrique's bill for this problem added up quickly. By the time he finally got a proper diagnosis, he had spent almost $3,000 and had missed several days of work. The lack of clarity in Enrique's initial complaint, and in the first MRI order cost Enrique time and money based on miscommunication.

In addition to the health organization, this story brings up another important player in the patient–provider interaction – the person or group who is responsible for payment of the expenses related to health care. Whether care is being paid for out of pocket, by private insurance, or a publicly financed program such as Medicare in the US, there will be constraints to what is allowed, based on financial concerns. The type of payment will dictate how much providers can charge for their services, which services they can offer, and how much of the cost for which the patient will be responsible. For example, procedures or medications that are deemed to be "experimental" may not be allowable. Insurance issues will need to be communicated to the patient before treatment begins.

Health care is expensive, and both patients and providers are seeking ways to minimize costs. In recent health-care reform debates, strategists argue that the process of making insurance payments should be modified. Smith (2009), the 2002 Nobel Laureate in economics, suggests that third-party insurance providers should make payments directly to patients, and then patients can pay providers directly for their services. This restructuring would allow for patient empowerment and enhance the relationship between patient and provider. While some economists argue that doctors and hospitals who are paid for each extra test will choose to conduct more care instead of better care, Don Boudreaux, an economics professor at George Mason University, suggests that the problem is not service fees but instead subsidized payments by third-party insurance providers (personal communication, November 9, 2009). Clearly, health-care payments are a hotly discussed topic in the health-care organization debate.

Seeing specialists is sometimes necessary, but it adds even more chaos to the chain of communication. Gaining appointments with specialists can take weeks or months, and when a patient does get in to see the doctor, he or she will need to make certain that the specialist has all the diagnostic tests and examination records from the primary physician and/or other specialists who have seen the patient.

All of these layers of health care create a difficult bureaucratic system that results in miscommunication, or even a total failure to communicate, among all the parties involved. The specialized nature and complexity of the health-care systems, however, make coordinated communication a vital part of successful care, especially when your condition is serious or ongoing. There is no room to let important information "fall through the cracks" during this progression.

In chapter 3, on patient characteristics, we examined the role of information management in patient participation in health care. In this chapter, we expand our look at how patients participate in health care by exploring a few organizational theories that can be used to make sense of patient–provider interactions.

Organizational socialization

A relevant organizational theory to describe how patients learn the rules of interaction with providers is organizational socialization (Jablin, 2001; Villagran and Hoffman, 2008). In cases when a patient is newly diagnosed with a chronic or ongoing condition, he or she is *socialized* into their treatment process. Diabetics, for example, may receive education about how to test their own sugar levels, or what to do in an emergency. Cancer patients are socialized into the cancer care process (Villagran and Hoffman, 2008). Some patients seek out information on blogs or Facebook groups about their condition and the facilities that deliver health care, but every patient has to eventually take part in face-to-face communication with health organizational members. These relationships set the stage for the health-care process.

Socialization of new patients by health-care providers is similar to being socialized into any other organization. It is helpful to think of a health issue as a new job, learning the ropes about what to do, and what not to do, to manage the job. Through interpersonal interactions with doctors, nurses, physical therapists, technicians, and other providers, information will be gained to make the new role go as smoothly as possible. There is often a new title or role associated with a new job, and here the new title is "patient," for example, a diabetes patient, an infertility patient, or an obes-ity patient. The title of this new "job" will provide a clearer path for building interactions and success in the care process.

Organizational socialization means gaining and managing relevant information about how to navigate through a health-care organization. It is the process of adjusting to a new role of self-advocate for effective health care. It involves learning about all the players on the health-care team. In the case of health-care organizations, the focus should be on adapting the care process or services of the organization to meet the needs of the individual patient. Research on organizational socialization generally refers to a three-step process, including an anticipatory phase, an entry phase, and an assimilation phase (Jablin, 2001; Villagran and Hoffman, 2008).

Patients in the *anticipatory phase* of socialization receive general information and form opinions about the larger health-care system and about specific relationships with trusted providers. The second phase, *organizational entry*, begins when a member first interacts with the health-care organization, and may include a general orientation delivered during the first few interactions. Patients find out about treatment protocols, and learn terminology related to their disease. Finally, the *assimilation* phase is when patients gain a clearer understanding of their role in health care, and gain a better picture of how each team member is allowed (or expected) to participate in health decision-making. The patient begins to make sense of what it means to be part of a health-care organization, in large part based on his or her interaction with a doctor, but all the providers in the health-care team interact to create a favorable or unfavorable relationship with the patient.

Patients in the *anticipatory phase* of socialization receive general information and form opinions about the larger health-care system, as well as about specific health organizations. Jablin (2001) explains that before entering an organization, individuals already have expectations and beliefs about how organizations such as the health-care system operate. A friend or family member may have recommended the physician or the hospital. Patients may perceive they know what to expect based on what they have watched on *Grey's Anatomy*. That information has an impact on whether patients choose to interact with an organization. Most research on the anticipatory phase has focused on where people get anticipatory messages

– educational institutions, the media, family and friends, or experiences with work.

In socializing members into health organizations, the anticipatory stage must be much more strategically constructed to convey a sense that the patient is a partner in their health care, and that the health organization is sensitive to the socio-demographic characteristics of the patient. This phase provides an opportunity for agency as the patient seeks out information and comes to understand the communication climate. Effective information sharing at this stage can help to create the underlying links so important to establishing a favorable decision-making climate. Second, effective communication and tailored information at this phase may create a more personal perception of the organization and enhance identification.

Messages in the anticipatory stage should also attempt to influence the decision-making climate. If members understand how making preferred health information management decisions helps them achieve a sense of agency and control over their situation, they are more likely to make those preferred choices. Messages in the anticipatory phase, for example, may link the shared value of family with decisions about whether to go forward with a particular treatment. By communicating in ways that identify shared values, agency of patients is enhanced because they have the information they need to feel more confident about their provider, as well as the larger health delivery system.

Miller and Jablin (1991) identified the entry phase as a key point for information seeking on the part of newcomers. They argue that newcomers' choices of information-seeking strategies are related to perceived social costs of information seeking. This is particularly important in socializing newcomers in health organizations because of the impact that information-seeking behaviors has been shown to have on health outcomes (Czaja et al., 2003). In order for newcomers in health organizations to use more direct information-seeking strategies, organizations need to communicate in ways that lower the perceived social cost. One way of doing this is to create an environment where seeking information and taking action on health issues does not violate closely held cultural or personal values.

Entry

During *entry* and *assimilation*, organizations focus on creating the favorable decision-making environment highlighted above. Part of being integrated into an organization means understanding how members are expected to make decisions, and sharing the values of the organization in making decisions. The entry phase begins when a member first interacts with the health-care organization. In traditional work organizations, this phase often entails an orientation program. In health organizations, it may include an orientation with a representative of the organization, as well as printed materials or videotapes.

Louis (1980) recognized that organizational newcomers require two specific types of information – task or role information, and cultural information. Likewise, in order to effectively socialize a new patient into the system within a doctor's office or in a hospital, information provided to the patient must address not only the specifics of a particular diagnosis, but also patient responsibilities related to long-term treatment and care. These messages will be most effective if they are based on shared values between the patient and the provider organization.

Patients should receive personalized socialization into health organizations based on their disease or health issue, their levels of social support, and their cultural background. The personalization of the system suggested in the anticipatory stage must be reinforced at entry. Fryer (1998) describes this process as "striving for purposeful self-determination, attempting to make sense of, initiate, influence, and cope with events in line with personal values, goals, and expectations of the future in a context of cultural norms, traditions, and past experiences" (p. 12). Table 9.1 outlines a variety of other strategies for personalizing socialization into health-care organizations for patients. For example, some specific strategies to increase personalization include identification of shared values, the use of collective pronouns like "we" and "our," and a consistent tone or unified voice across organizational documents (Cheney, 1983). This reinforces the idea that health-care decisions will be made in a collaborative manner.

Sense-making

Karl Weick (1969) describes how organizations do not really exist outside human interaction, but rather are constructed by continued human interaction. In other words, a patient's unique health-care experience is based on a person's unique medical condition, social and psychological state, and financial resources. Communication about health-care experiences is organized into a story, or narrative, that is written based on the interplay among each of these three factors. Just as a health-care narrative is the first part of each medical visit, the narrative is the running story of the health care received and the organization and providers who delivered it.

Weick's model is built on several primary ideas from socio-cultural evolutionary theory, information theory, and systems theory (Kreps, 2007; Kreps, Villagran and Zhao, forthcoming). Each theory offers a specific piece to a puzzle that becomes what we experience as a health-care delivery system. First, patients vary, and adapt to, changes in their social and cultural environments. Patients vary their approaches with doctors based on what they perceived to be effective in the past. People often devise communicative strategies before their medical encounters by playing out the anticipated scene in their head. If something a patient said elicited the intended response from a provider, the patient will retain that information for later use. If a patient tells a provider a story, or a joke, to help explain a health issue, the patient will retain the response to that communicative strategy, whether or not the provider laughs at the joke.

Weick's interpretation of the role of information was focused upon how

Table 9.2 Strategies to personalize patient socialization in health-care provider organizations

Organizational elements	Personalization for patients
Organizational structure	Inclusive governance with community advisory board.
	Opportunities for informal interpersonal contact with providers such as provider-sponsored support groups.
	Policies and procedures to require a balance between task and relational communication.
Materials for patients and employees	Physical environment includes décor, signage and graphics written in the appropriate tone for the specific patient group.
	All printed and AV materials make use of culturally competent language and shared values, as well as inclusive ("we" and "our") language.
	Distribution of staff bios to patients.
Staff diversity	Representative staff for diverse patient populations on all work shifts.
Staff training and development	Regular team-building exercises.
	Patient communication seminars.
	Evaluation of employee learning outcomes.
Interpreter services	All medical visits include qualified interpreter.
	Interpreters trained in language and culture.
	No family member interpreters.
	Interpreters available for telephone consultations.
Tracking system for patients	Patient satisfaction assessment throughout health-care process.
	Navigator/patient advocate program for patients from underserved groups.

Source: OMH (2003)

to share and retain information, and in health-care interactions this is especially important. To avoid confusion or miscommunication, patients seek out the most effective channels to talk to their providers, and those channels often come from the health organization. Health-care organizations exist to achieve certain health-related tasks (such as diagnosis, testing, treatment) by building certain relationships (between patients and providers, and among providers). Interdependence among members of the health-care team creates a larger system where every member must do his or her part for the patients. For example, if a patient has a particular disease, he will need a general practitioner or internist, a nurse, a host of different specialists for the specific health concern, a person to do the intake for the visits, and a team of technicians and other professionals to give tests, take blood, do X-rays, and help with payment issues. No one member of the system can provide improved health for the patient, but, as a whole, the delivery team will operate as a team with a unique hierarchical structure, to deliver health care to the patient. Feedback among members of the health-care team will be used to monitor the process of the patient, and the success of the system.

The process of *sense-making* for a patient occurs based on interpretation of actions and responses of those in the health-care interaction. After a diagnosis, there is a need for information exchange and shared meaning creation that in turn generates a new organizational structure. An organization, according to Weick, is really a process of bringing order out of chaos and organizing a new reality for the patient.

The final aspect of Weick's model of organizing that directly relates to the way patients experience health care through their relationships with providers is *equivocality,* which is very similar to the concept of uncertainty in other theories we have already discussed. Patients and providers often must cope with very complex situations, and equivocality must be met with equivocality. In other words, there are not usually easy answers to difficult or complex questions. When patients feel frustrated by the long, jargon-filled answers they may receive to a question, it may be the doctors' attempt to be as accurate as possible even though that means the answer has multiple parts and areas that can be confusing. To handle equivocal (or uncertain) situations, doctors should seek as many cues as possible from the patient about his/her information needs. If the patient is really just looking for a clear simple answer, doctors should react with very simple responses that have been effective with patients in the past. As organizational members, patients and providers make sense of uncertainty in their health-care system in an effort to avoid distortion and maximize the flow of information.

Symbolic convergence theory

When patients feel a lack of trust about certain health-care organizations, they will often share stories about other patients who have had bad experiences in the facility. For example, a medical-testing facility near a college campus might be known for paying students to be participants in dangerous medical experiments. Whether the experiments are dangerous is not the issue; instead, the important point is that students believe the health organization is not trustworthy.

There is an urban legend that exists in some communities about a hospital that is commonly referred to as the place where patients go in but never come out. The actual name of the hospital is rarely used, but when people refer to it, everyone knows a person, who knows a person, who went into the hospital for a routine procedure and never came out. The hospital is usually called *The Hospital of Last Resort*. The story is told in reference to a variety of hospitals in a variety of regions of the country. Part of the urban legend among residents near these hospitals is that the facility is a cover for a secret government program that conducts tests on patients without their knowledge.

As a result, some patients are skeptical about the advice from providers who work there. Other patients talk openly about their mistrust of providers and test results performed in the hospital. The result of a shared fantasy, or urban legend, about the hospital is that many of the provider–patient interactions are negatively impacted by false information. Patients are less satisfied with their care, more likely to seek a second opinion, and less likely to adhere to treatment recommendations because they perceive the organization to be of poor quality, or even blatantly sinister. In every case, patients feel more concerned about receiving treatment from the hospital because it has a bad reputation in the community. Word of mouth is essential. In fact, over 50 percent of people rely on personal recommendations from family and friends when choosing a primary health-care provider (Tu and Lauer, 2008).

Even if people do not know a hospital like the one described here, they may have heard of a doctor who is unscrupulous, or they may have received false or exaggerated information about what it's like to have a particular disease. We view our health and illness based in part on the organizations, the structures, and the systems through which we receive care. When you make your appointment, you may choose to avoid "that doctor" about whom you have heard terrible stories. You may have even contributed to the "legend" of a doctor or health-care facility by sharing your own experiences in a slightly dramatic way. For example, when you go in the hospital the food is never exceptionally good, but it is also not usually quite as bad as the stories you might tell about your meals. Was it really green? Was it really moving on its own? Did you really see bugs crawling out of it? Real or imagined, fantasy themes shape our interactions. Ernest Bormann's symbolic convergence theory (SCT; 1972) is a description of the dynamic process of sharing group fantasies. Patients and providers interact within a larger health-care organization and health-care system that may exhibit characteristics Bormann refers to as aspects *of fantasy*, emotion, and rhetoric in the creation of symbolic reality. If medical encounters are impacted by the context and culture within which they occur, then the symbolic reality of what it is to give and receive health care is shaped by the stories about patients, organizational rules, structures, and leadership of the organization.

SCT is a group theory that focuses on the message as the unit of analysis, emphasizing the communicative processes in which individuals converge their fantasies, meanings, and symbolic realities. The manner by which people come to share a common reality or world-view is the premise behind SCT. By investigating the talk that humans share with each other, and exploring how they collectively construct a communal view of health-care systems, SCT provides a potential framework for thinking about how our views of health care in general can shape our interactions with providers.

Meanings of events and messages, emotions we face during the process, and motives for recommendations or treatment options are viewed as part of a larger protocol or system. Symbols provide a means by which people can express shared feelings, emotions and fears that are related but not always identical. For example, if my fear of blood is manifested emotionally every time I see a needle, I am less likely to visit a clinic or be friendly when I do have to get a shot. Personal emotions can be expanded to a single group emotion if like-minded patients share their feelings. The stories and experiences resulting from these emotions are expanded through *fantasy chains*.

Fantasy chains begin with individual expressions of a personal fantasy, emotion, or fear. That fantasy is then established, and develops and grows as it is shared among other patients with a similar disease type, or among people who use the same health-care facility. The health-care organization becomes the symbol of the fantasy, but the provider–patient relationship is where the actual impact of the fantasy is experienced. We shape our communication based on our views of the world, both real and imagined. Patients who believe their care is sub-standard or experimental will not interact with their care team in the same way as patients who trust their providers. The fantasy theme is created to deal with fear or emotion, but it fosters even more fear and emotion as it grows larger. Every urban legend has the capacity to make us behave in irrational ways. Fantasy themes about health-care organizations impact the patients and providers in irrational ways as well.

Health-care team communication

Although a hospital may be viewed as a central organizational structure for health-care delivery, patients typically interact with members of a variety of organizations during the care process. Until the last century, medical teams or groups of providers were almost non-existent (Lammers et al., 2003). When the Mayo brothers opened their clinic in Rochester, Minnesota, they included a group of providers who sought to care for the railroad workers who came to their area (Lammers et al., 2003). Mayo's concept that "No one is big enough to be independent of others" led to the development of one of the world's first private group practices of medicine (Mayoclinic.org). A hospital is just one type of group practice where care occurs. Others include doctors' offices, specialty clinics, diagnostic technology centers, and surgery centers. The fact that health care almost never occurs in just one physical location for a patient requires a concerted effort to develop and coordinate communication between and among all parties who deliver care for that patient. Similarly, patients often think in terms of one doctor or health-care provider who is in charge of their care. The old model of a family doctor who is present from birth until death rarely exists in today's world. In reality, it is rare to receive all health care from just one provider, especially over a lifetime.

Ideally, the health-care team works together to make decisions and provider-coordinated care. In fact, team cohesion has been linked to improved performance (i.e., Chang and Bordia, 2001), so patient health outcomes can be improved when a cohesive team delivers high-quality care. Cohesive health delivery teams use multiple channels for frequent interactions about patient care. Sometimes the communication among team members is a regular part of the day, but sometimes the amount and quality of communication about patients is limited by time and conflicting schedules. Writing notations in a patient's chart is one of the most common channels of communication between members of a health-care team. Instead of talking to each other in face-to-face communication, written messages among team members are intended to create continuity of care. Patients' charts include information about their day-to-day vital statistics, as well as their diagnosis and treatment history. Although some organizations are moving toward electronic medical records, handwritten, paper charts are still the most common form of patient records. Busy providers often mistakenly write incorrect information in the charts. Below is a sample of humorous notes found in patients' paper charts.

> The lab test indicated abnormal lover function.
> She stated that she had been constipated for most of her life until 1989 when she got a divorce.
> The patient was in his usual state of good health until his airplane ran out of gas and crashed.
> She is numb from her toes down.
> On the second day the knee was better and on the third day it had completely disappeared.
> The patient is tearful and crying constantly. She also appears to be depressed.
> Discharge status: Alive but without permission. (Lederer, 2000: 64–8)

Even though many physicians and surgeons work long, irregular hours, finding time to communicate about patients with other health-care providers takes a back seat to communicating directly with patients and their families. In health organizations there are several characteristics of effective health-care teams to look out for as a patient. It is completely acceptable for a patient to ask important questions about the team providing his or her care.

The following points show some important issues to consider.

What is this health-care team's collective level of experience?
Teams will probably include physicians and surgeons with years of experience with patients, and some residents, interns, or medical students who have significantly less experience.

What are the normal patterns of interaction of this team?
This question includes regular hours when team members might be available to meet with patients and family members. Also, are there formal leaders in the group to whom patients should direct important questions about their care? Do certain team members have specialized information about which patients should be aware? Sometimes just knowing whom the correct person is to ask questions can improve a person's ability to get timely answers and ensure his or her concerns are made clear to the right audience.

When a patient suspects his or her team may not be communicating with each other on a regular basis, it becomes especially important to know the best time and to whom questions should be directed. Teams that meet very early in the morning, for example, such as those who work in hospitals, may not communicate with each other again for the rest of the day. Making sure questions are put to the right person in advance of that morning meeting can mean the difference between getting an answer on that day or waiting 24 hours until the team meets again.

Is your health-care team diverse based on their cultural, social, or socio-demographic backgrounds, and in relation to your own socio-demographic characteristics?
Some patients feel more comfortable with a provider who is of the same sex, or about the same age, or from the same cultural background as the patient. Health-care teams are often comprised of persons from a variety of backgrounds, but as a patient it can be beneficial to understand which team members might identify most closely with oneself.

Do members of the health-care team appear to be satisfied with their jobs?
Often high job satisfaction, or a feeling that a job is meaningful and rewarding, can lead to less turnover, less burnout, and more cohesion in work teams. If a health-care team has a high degree of job satisfaction, the members are more likely to treat patients with a high level of respect. Coordination among team members is also more likely to occur on a regular basis because the team will probably have worked together for a longer period of time.

Do you witness any conflict between members of your health-care team?
Conflict might be harsh words about a missing chart, an overlooked request for assistance, or an unreturned page or phone call. Team members who exhibit signs of conflict are less likely to have consistent, meaningful communication with each other about a patient's case and concerns. In this situation, it is important for a patient to repeat key questions or problems to each team member as he or she sees them. It cannot be assumed that team members are sharing patient information with each other. In addition, when information is shared, it is more likely that misunderstandings or reframing of a patient's concerns will occur. Conflict in health organizations can occur without impacting patients, but when a health-care team seems to exhibit consistent conflict or harsh words to or about each other, as a patient it is important to avoid being caught in the middle. It can help

if a patient is honest with providers about any conflict he or she witnesses, and to let them know if it makes him or her uncomfortable, while reporting extreme concerns to leaders of the health organization.

Although as a patient it is not usually possible to completely change the health delivery team based on perceived lack of effective communication, if patients ask themselves these questions it can help reveal potential *cracks*, or places where information could be lost or misrepresented.

Provider–patient interactions in hospice organizations

As mentioned, a hospital may be viewed as a central organizational structure for health-care delivery, but patients will interact with members of a variety of organizations. The health-care process can include a hospital, doctors' offices, specialty clinics, diagnostic technology centers, and surgery centers. The variety of locations means it is important for a patient to develop and coordinate communication between and among all parties. One especially unique health organization based on the structure and function of communication is the hospice. Although hospice organizations often work in concert with other health-care team members, the goal of hospice makes communication in hospice environments distinctive. Hospice organizations are designed specifically to support terminally ill patients and their families. Some hospice organizations are housed within hospitals, some are in stand-alone buildings, and sometimes hospice team members visit patients in their own homes. Regardless of the physical location of a hospice, the organizational goals are to improve the quality of a patient's final days through an organized approach to end-of-life.

Hospice care is typically defined as end-of-life care provided by health professionals and volunteers who give medical, psychological, and spiritual support. The goal of the care is to help people who are dying have peace, comfort, and dignity. The caregivers try to control pain and other symptoms so a person can remain as alert and comfortable as possible. Hospice programs also provide services to support a patient's family (<http://www.nlm.nih.gov/medlineplus/hospicecare.html>). Hospices are becoming an increasingly common and mainstream part of medical care. Over the past two decades, hospice organizations have become more prevalent in response to the desire of most patients with serious, incurable diseases to die at home. Dying at home is associated with greater satisfaction by bereaved family members (Ratner, Norlander, and McSteen, 2001). Individuals are increasingly concerned with the importance of dying with dignity and desire to experience a more meaningful, comfortable, and supportive end-of-life with loved ones (Lynn, 2001). Trends indicate that hospices are becoming an attractive alternative to dying in a clinical setting, but only a fraction of patients with an option of hospice choose to participate. Physicians and nurses must communicate more openly with patients and families about the benefits of end-of-life care to maximize use of supportive hospice services in the difficult time of facing death (Hospice Association of America, 2009).

Although hospices usually provide end-of-life care to patients at home rather than in hospitals, the majority of individuals in this country still die in hospitals and nursing homes (von Gunten, 2002). Most hospice care takes place in the patient's home, although more and more in-patient hospice facilities are becoming available. In-patient hospice facilities are helpful for patients who do not have family members or other loved ones to care for them. Hospice staff members do not usually serve as primary caregivers for a patient enrolled in a home hospice program. A family member is typically the primary caregiver and he or she often helps make decisions for the terminally ill individual. Members of the hospice staff support the family caregiver by making regular visits to assess the patient and provide additional care or other services. Hospice staff workers are usually available to patients and family members 24 hours a day, seven days a week.

The hospice physician and/or nurses are usually responsible for making decisions about increases and decreases in pain medication and the treatment of other physical symptoms, although pain and symptoms are usually monitored on a daily basis by the family caregiver. Hospice staff members provide family caregivers with training in pain and symptom monitoring as well as a host of other caregiver tasks, and the hospice program provides all medications and supplies needed to care for the patient (National Hospice and Palliative Care Organization, 2009). Various aspects and issues of death and dying are taken on by the hospice team, who also tend to assist the patient and their family members with the emotional, psychosocial, and spiritual aspects surrounding death. Following the death of a hospice patient, bereavement services and counseling are also available to loved ones for a year (Hospice Foundation of America, 2010).

Most insurance plans do not adequately cover services needed for quality end-of-life care (Raphael, Ahrens, and Fowler, 2001). Outside of hospice organizations, there are few ways that people can be reimbursed for these types of services. One of the reasons that insurance plans are reluctant to cover end-of-life care is due to the fact that some diseases, such as cancer, progress to late stages where people experience multiple physical symptoms that can be expensive to treat. Most insurance plans currently do not recognize, or only provide limited reimbursement for, services that meet the psychosocial needs of patients, such as patient counseling, counseling for family members, or other services that do not deal with physical health (Reb, 2003).

Cultural barriers to hospices exist and are worth noting. Most hospice organizations do a wonderful job of addressing psychosocial concerns, but most continue to adopt a conventional Western perspective of health care. Studies indicate that individuals with lower socioeconomic status are less likely to be referred to hospice programs (Grande, McKerral, and Todd, 2002). Research indicates that black/minority ethnic populations are referred to hospice less often than White populations (Karim, Bailey, and Tunna, 2000). Poulson (1998) identified several salient cultural issues to be considered during end-of-life care, including the possible need for translators, varying religious traditions, differing communication patterns, diverse social customs, familial hierarchies, and death rituals. Hospices have come a long way in the US health-care system and are for the most part very positive additions to end-of-life health care, but cultural barriers and issues remain understudied.

Despite vast improvements in public health and health care in the US and worldwide over the last century, we still have a long way to go in terms of making our society and the world a healthier place. The United States spent $2.2 trillion on health care in 2007, which computes to $7,421 per person. This is nearly twice the average cost spent by other nations on health care. If this trend continues, the Congressional Budget Office estimates that, by 2025, one in every four dollars of the economic budget will go to health care (The White House, 2009). The rising costs of health insurance and health services are likely to continue having a substantial impact on consumers in the coming years. Health-care organizations are always trying to find innovative ways to reduce the cost of health-care services (which ultimately influences the cost of health-care insurance). Many costly problems, such as high provider turnover rates, are often related to communication problems. As a result, health communication researchers have developed interventions designed to ameliorate these problems and to reduce costs that are ultimately passed along to consumers. However, much more research is needed to discover how communication interventions can be used to make health-care organizations more efficient, helpful, and satisfying for patients.

Conclusion

In this chapter we have highlighted some of the organizational issues that impact provider–patient communication. There is no question that organizational structures impact the way we access and experience health care, and the options for care available to patients are driven in large part by the type of health-care organization to which they belong. Patients may hear stories that affect their views of the health-care system and then alter their interactions with providers based on those views. Patients who desire to be part of their health care must exhibit a sense of agency by acting and interacting as a co-equal member in their own health care. Physicians are highly trained experts with a wealth of information about disease and illness, and patients are experts on their own fears, levels of social support, tolerance for pain, and need for information. Together, providers and patients can negotiate within health-care organizations to find the most appropriate health-care solutions for the patient.

Discussion Questions for Evaluating the Health Organization

Navigating the complex system of the health organization can pose challenges for patients. These organizations function with multiple levels and doctors involved, which opens up possibilities for miscommunication among groups and individuals. In order for patients to ensure that they receive the best care from their health-care team, it is helpful to ask specific questions of team members.

Are you affiliated with a specific health-care center or hospital where I will need to go for treatment?

Do you often work with other providers in my health-care team?

How often do you speak with other health-care team members?

How is my medical information distributed/shared between team members?

How many providers are included in my health-care team?

What level of experience does each member have in relation to my condition?

Can I have the opportunity to meet my individual team members before treatment begins?

PART V

PATIENT AND PROVIDER INTERACTION
EPILOGUE

10 Patient and Provider Interaction: Epilogue

It is important to recognize that health-care delivery mechanisms are changing during the twenty-first century and we all need to adapt in the best and most efficient, compassionate ways possible. It takes a global village to truly achieve the best health decisions and outcomes for all.

We hope we have offered evidence-based, insightful analyses and descriptions of how to achieve more fruitful health-care interactions that ultimately lead to better and more informed health decisions and outcomes. Patient and provider interaction and the study of health communication have generated intense national and international interest over the last decade. There is a desperate need for health-care leaders who possess strong interpersonal, observational, analytical, and management skills, as well as complementary emotional skills that demonstrate compassion for the uncertainties that patients and loved ones are experiencing. Such skills are needed not only for assessing effectiveness of treatments, practitioner and organizational performance, but also to promote modern attitudes and appropriate, much needed positive changes in clinical behavior that will benefit all involved. Multiple messages must be given to patients (e.g., written, oral, phone, text, email). Providers should be asking patients what messages they prefer receiving and patients should politely remind providers and staff members how they can best receive delicate health information. Similarly, it is time for patients and health-care consumers to step up while remaining mindful of the many competing responsibilities that providers may be dealing with at any given time (e.g., time constraints, organizational and management issues, insurance problems, staffing and personnel issues, technical and mechanical issues, as well as financial issues that impact the systems within a practice). Patient choice is key, but appropriate, accessible, relevant, and accurate health information, available during patient and provider interaction, must exist for patients to have the tools to make the best choices possible.

In this book, we have attempted to provide accessible, accurate, relevant and (at times) entertaining evidence-based health information that can provide guidelines to navigate the complex health-care environment. Understanding high-quality, credible, accessible health information is a crucial component of health-care delivery and decision-making. Such interactions are two-way and are best achieved through committed providers *and* patients, family members, and friends involved.

The often-repeated phrase, [health] "information is power," is absolutely true in the health-care environment. Providers need accurate and accessible health information from the patients in order to give the best care possible. Patients need accurate and accessible health information so they can talk with their providers and loved ones, then make the best health decisions that fit their life in terms of time commitment and barriers, transportation commitment and barriers, financial commitment and barriers, social commitment and barriers, and so on. Health-care interactions are not a panacea, but are complementary to achieving the best health goals and outcomes possible. As health communicators, we can assist with the achievement of the best possible life from a health messages perspective. Ultimately, it is all about the relationship between patients and providers and all involved in the health-care system. We must be kind and compassionate toward one another and not be constantly worried about lawyers and insurance companies, and pages and pages of informed consent forms that may prevent the best care possible.

How can it be that in the twenty-first century we see signs on hospital buildings telling us that if we enter we might expose ourselves to cancer-producing agents? These signs must look ridiculous to everyone but the people who actually decided to put them there. In the end, we must reflect on the times when a handshake meant something, one's word meant something – this is the American society and health-care system that will best serve its people. Being true to our word ensures a more positive experience.

It is our responsibility (whether serving in a provider or patient role) to be true and authentic as we talk with each other – to care about building a relationship of sorts. It is ultimately through the relationships we build and maintain with people that we will achieve the best care possible.

We hope this book helps in the accomplishment of a substantial quality of life, full of joy and cheerfulness in all that is experienced, whether one is a patient, loved one, or provider. Keeping in touch with other interests and people outside of the health-care environment, if only for short spurts of time, adds to the quality of all other aspects of life. Doing one thing for ourselves each day – whether it is an hour of walking, running, tae kwon do, meditation, yoga, boot camp, total body sculpting, reading, massage, praying, cooking, shopping, etc. – provides support and balance in our lives.

Each of us knows our own self better than anyone, so keeping in touch with ourselves and remaining true to ourselves and those around us every day ensures we will not give up who we are or lose our personal goals in life – even when people try to take them away. In these ways, we can discover the beauty in each phase of our life journey. This is sometimes difficult to do, but it is important to continue to see the beauty even when it seems to be hiding at times.

Though it may seem that the health-care situation is impossible and the challenges are overwhelming and nothing can be done, opportunities exist to further extend and develop health-care practice, delivery systems, understanding each other from spiritual and cultural perspectives and their relationship to health outcomes and well-being. We hope that providers and patients can commit to creating and maintaining stronger relationships during challenging times of uncertainty by utiliz-ing the principles discussed in *Patient and Provider Interaction*. We are all challenged to do so in an often cumbersome, rigid health-care culture, but if we remain cheerful, sensitive, compassionate, dedicated, and flexible, while connecting with each other, it can be done – and it will be easier than everyone thinks!

References

Accreditation Council for Graduate Medical Education (1999). *Outcome Project*. Available from: <http://www.acgme.org/outcome/comp/refCom1.asp>.

Afifi, W. A., and Guerrero, L. K. (2000). Motivations underlying topic avoidance in close relationships. In S. Petronio (ed.), *Balancing the Secrets of Private Disclosures* (pp. 165–80). Mahwah, NJ: Erlbaum.

Afifi, W. A., and Weiner, J. L. (2004). Toward a theory of motivated information management. *Communication Theory*, 14: 167–90.

Al-Deen, H. S. N. (1997). Preface. In H. S. N. Al-Deen (ed.), *Cross-cultural Communication and Aging in the United States* (pp. xi–xiii). Mahwah, NJ: Lawrence Erlbaum.

Alba, J. W., and Marmorstein, H. (1987). The effects of frequency knowledge on consumer decision making. *The Journal of Consumer Research*, 14: 14–25.

Albrecht, T. L., Burleson, B. R., and Goldsmith, D. (1994). Supportive communication. In M. L. Knapp and G. R. Miller (eds), *Handbook of Interpersonal Communication* (2nd edn, pp. 419–49). Newbury Park, CA: Sage.

Albrecht, T. L., and Goldsmith, D. J. (2003). Social support, social networks, and health. In T. L. Thompson et al. (eds), *Handbook of Health Communication* (pp. 263–84). Mahwah, NJ: Lawrence Erlbaum Associates.

Allen, R. S., Haley, W. E., Small, B. J., McMillan, S. C. (2002). Pain reports by older hospice cancer patients and family caregivers: The role of cognitive functioning. *The Gerontologist*, 42: 507–14.

Allport, G. W. (1954). *The Nature of Prejudice*. Reading, MA: Addison-Wesley.

Alzheimer's Disease Education and Referral Center (2007). *Connections*, 15. Available at: <http://www.nia.nih.gov/NR/rdonlyres/73382FBD-A107-4E15-9701-85D64854B4ED/7836/Connections_v15n12.pdf>.

American Association of Retired Persons (AARP) (2009). *Caregiving in the U. S. 2009*. Available at: <http://www.aarp.org/research/surveys/care/ltc/hc/articles/ caregiving_09.html>.

American Society for Quality. (2005, February). *Healthcare*. Available at: <http://www.kff.org/kaiserpolls/7209.cfm>.

American Society of Clinical Oncology. (2009, May 18). Caring for the whole patient. Available at: <http://www.cancer.net/patient/Coping/Caring+for+the+Whole+Patient>.

Amir, Y. (1976). The role of intergroup contact in change of prejudice and race relations. In P. A. Katz (ed.), *Toward the Elimination of Prejudice* (pp. 245–80). New York: Pergamon.

Anderson, J. O., and Martin, P. G. (2003). Narratives and healing: Exploring one family's stories of cancer survivorship. *Health Communication*, 15(2): 133–43.

Anderson, K. H. (1998). The relationship between family sense of coherence and family quality of life after illness diagnosis. In H. I. McCubbin, and T. Elizabeth (eds), *Stress, Coping, and Health in Families: Sense of Coherence and Resiliency* (pp. 47–55). New York: Sage Publications.

Anderson, N. B. (1989). Racial differences in stress-induced cardiovascular reactivity and hypertension: Current status and substantive issues. *Psychological Bulletin*, 105: 89–105.

Anderson, W. G., Arnold, R. M., Angus, D. C., and Bryce, C. L. (2009). Passive decision-making preference is associated with anxiety and depression in relatives of patients in the intensive care unit. *Journal of Critical Care,* 24: 249–54.

Andrews, S. C. (2001). Caregiver burden and symptom distress in people with cancer receiving hospice care. *Oncology Nursing Forum,* 28: 1469–74.

Aneshensel, C. S., and Stone, J. D. (1982). Stress and depression: A test of the buffering model of social support. *Archives of General Psychiatry,* 39: 1392–6.

Antze, P. (1976). The role of ideologies in peer psychotherapy organizations: Some theoretical considerations and three case studies. *Journal of Applied Behavioral Science,* 12: 323–46.

Aoki, Y., et al. (1997). Significance of informed consent and truth-telling for quality of life in terminal cancer patients. *Radiation Medicine,* 15: 133–5.

Armstrong, L., and Jenkins, S. (2000). *It's Not about the Bike: My Journey Back to Life.* New York: Putnam Publishing.

Arntson, P., and Droge, D. (1987). Social support in self-help groups: The role of communication in enabling perceptions of control. In T. L. Albrecht, M. B. Adelman, and Associates (eds), *Communicating Social Support* (pp. 148–71). Newbury Park, CA: Sage.

Aroian, J. F., Meservey, P. M., and Crockett, J. (1996). Developing nurse leaders for today and tomorrow: Part 1, Foundations of leadership in practice. *Journal of Nursing Administration,* 26: 18–26.

Aroian, J. F., Patsdaughter, C. A., and Wyszynski, M. E. (2000). DONs in long-term care facilities: Contemporary roles, current credentials, and educational needs. *Nursing Economics,* 18: 149–56.

Arora, N., and McHorney, C. (2000). Patient preferences for medical decision making. *Medical Care,* 38(3): 335–41.

Arrington, M. (2000). Thinking inside the box: On identity, sexuality, prostate cancer, and social support. *Journal of Aging and Identity,* 5 (3): 151–8.

Aspden, P., and Katz, J. (2001). Assessments of quality of health care information and referrals to physicians: A nationwide survey. In R. E. Rice and J. Katz (eds), *The Internet and Health Communication. Experiences and Expectations* (pp. 107–19). Thousand Oaks, CA: Sage Publications.

Aspden, P., Katz, J. E., and Bemis, A. (2001). Use of the Internet for professional purposes: A survey of New Jersey physicians. In R. E. Rice, and J. E. Katz (eds), *The Internet and Health Communication: Experiences and Expectations* (pp. 107–20).

Ayanian, J. Z., and Cleary, P. D. (1999). Perceived risk of heart disease and cancer among cigarette smokers. *Journal of the American Medical Association,* 281: 1019.

Aylor, B. A. (2003). Maintaining long-distance relationships. In D. J. Canary and M. Dainton (eds), *Maintaining Relationships through Communication* (pp. 127–39). Mahwah, NJ: Erlbaum.

Azjen, I., and Fishbein, M. (2000). Attitudes and the attitude–behavior relation: Reasoned and automatic processes. In W. Stroebe and M. Hewstone (eds), *European Review of Social Psychology* (Vol. 11, pp. 1–33). New York: Wiley.

Babrow, A. S. (1992). Communication and problematic integration: Understanding diverging probability and value, ambiguity, ambivalence, and impossibility. *Communication Theory,* 2: 95–130.

Babrow, A. S. (1995). Communication and problematic integration: Milan Kundera's "Lost Letters" in The Book of Laughter and Forgetting. *Communication Monographs,* 62: 283–300.

Babrow, A. S. (2001). Uncertainty, value, communication, and problematic integration. *Journal of Communication,* 51: 553–73.

Babrow, A. S., Kasch, C. R., and Ford, L. A. (1998). The many meanings of uncertainty in illness: Toward a systematic accounting. *Health Communication,* 10(1): 1–23.

Back, A., et al. (2007). Efficacy of communication skills training for giving bad news and discussing transitions to palliative care. *Archives of Internal Medicine*, 167(5): 453–60.

Baile, W., Buckman, R., Schipira, L., and Parker, P. (2006). Breaking bad news: More than just guidelines. *Journal of Clinical Oncology*, 24(19): 3217.

Baile, W., et al. (2000). SPIKES – A six-step protocol for delivering bad news: Application to the patient with cancer. *Oncologist*, 5(4): 302–11.

Baillie, L. (2007). Family caregiving when relationships are poor. In I. Paoletti (ed.), *Family Caregiving for Older Disabled People* (pp. 127–49). New York: Nova Science Publishers.

Bakas, T., Lewis, R. R., and Parsons, J. (2001). Caregiving tasks among family caregivers of patients with lung cancer. *Oncology Nursing Forum*, 28: 847–54.

Bakas, T., et al. (2002). Needs, concerns, strategies, and advice of stroke caregivers the first six months after discharge. *Journal of Neuroscience Nursing*, 34(5): 242–51.

Baker, D. W., et al. (1996). The health care experience of patients with low literacy. *Archives of Family Medicine*, 5(6): 329–34.

Baker, D. W., et al. (1999). Development of a brief test to measure functional health literacy. *Patient Education and Counseling*, 38: 33–42.

Baker, D. W., et al. (2002). Functional health literacy and the risk of hospital admission among Medicare managed care enrollees. *American Journal of Public Health*, 92(8): 1278–83.

Baker, D. W., et al. (2007). Health literacy and mortality among elderly persons. *Archives of Internal Medicine*, 167: 1503–9.

Baldassar, L., and Baldock. C. V. (2000). Linking migration and family studies: Transnational migrants and the care of ageing parents. In B. Agozino (ed.), *Theoretical and Methodological Issues in Migration Research: Interdisciplinary, Intergenerational and International Perspectives* (pp. 61–89). Aldershot: Ashgate.

Baldassar, L., Wilding, R., and Baldock, C. (2007). Long-distance caregiving: Transnational families and the provision of aged care. In I. Paoletti (ed.), *Family Caregiving for Older Disabled People* (pp. 201–27). New York: Nova Science Publishers.

Baldock, C. V. (1999). The ache of frequent farewells. In M. Poole and S. Feldman (eds), *A Certain Age: Women Growing Older* (pp. 182–92). St Leonards, Australia: Allen and Unwin.

Baldock, C. V. (2000). Migrants and their parents: Caregiving from a distance. *Journal of Family Issues*, 21: 205–24.

Ballard-Reisch, D. (1996). Coping with alienation, fear, and isolation: The disenfranchisement of adolescents with cancer and their families. In E. Berlin Ray (ed.). *Communication and Disenfranchisement: Social Health Issues and Implications* (pp. 185–208). Mahwah, NJ: Lawrence Erlbaum Association, Publishers.

Ballieux, R. E., and Heijen, C. J. (1989). Stress and the immune response. In H. Weiner, I. Floring, R. Murison, and D. Hellhammer (eds), *Frontiers of Stress Research* (pp. 51–5). Toronto, Canada: Huber.

Baltes, P. B. (1987). Theoretical propositions of life-span developmental psychology: On the dynamics of growth and decline. *Developmental Psychology*, 23: 611–26.

Baltes, P. B., and Baltes, M. M. (1990). Psychological perspectives on successful aging: The model of selective optimization with compensation. In P. B. Baltes and M. M. Baltes (eds), *Successful Aging: Perspectives from the Behavioral Sciences* (pp. 1–34). New York: Cambridge University Press.

Bandura, A. (1977). *Social Learning Theory.* Englewood Cliffs, NJ: Prentice Hall.

Bandura, A. (1989). Perceived self-efficacy in the exercise of control over AIDS infection. In V. M. Mays, G. W. Albee, and S. S. Schneider (eds), *Primary Prevention of AIDS: Psychological Approaches* (pp. 128–41). Newbury Park, CA: Sage.

Bandura, A. (1997). *Self-efficacy: The Exercise of Control.* New York: W. H. Freeman.

Banker, B. S., and Gaertner, S. L. (1998). Achieving stepfamily harmony: An intergroup-relations approach. *Journal of Family Psychology*, 12: 310–25.

Banks, A. T., Zimmerman, H. J., Ishak, K. G., and Harter, J. G. (1995). Diclofenac-associated hepatotoxicity: Analysis of 180 cases reported to the Food and Drug Administration as adverse reactions. *Hepatology*, 22(3): 820–7.

Banks, S., et al. (1995). The effects of message framing on mammography utilization. *Health Psychology*, 14: 178–84.

Banks, S. P., Ge, G., and Baker, J. (1991). Intercultural encounters and miscommunication. In: J. Coupland, H. Giles, and M. Wiemann (eds). *Miscommunication and Problematic Talk*. London: Sage.

Baquet, C. R., and Hunter, C. P. (1995). Patterns in minority and special populations. In P. Greenwald, B. Kramer, and D. L. Weed (eds) *Cancer Prevention and Control* (pp. 23–36). New York: Marcel Dekker.

Barach, P., and Small, S. D. (2000). Reporting and preventing medical mishaps: Lessons from non-medical near miss reporting systems. *British Medical Journal*, 320: 759–63.

Barbee, A. P. (1990). Interactive coping: The cheering-up process in close relationships. In S. Duck and R. Silver (eds), *Personal Relationships and Social Support* (pp. 46–65). Newbury Park, CA: Sage.

Barclay, S., et al. (2003). Care for the dying: How well prepared are general practitioners? A questionnaire study in Wales. *Palliative Medicine*, 17: 27–39.

Barnes, M. D., et al. (2003). Measuring the relevance of evaluation criteria among health information seekers on the Internet. *Journal of Health Psychology*, 8: 71–82.

Barnes, M. K., and Duck, S. (1994). Everyday communicative contexts for social support. In B. R. Burleson, T. L. Albrecht, and I. G. Sarason (eds), *Communication of Social Support: Messages, Interactions, Relationships, and Community* (pp. 175–94). Thousand Oaks, CA: Sage.

Barr, M. S. (2008). The need to test the patient-centered medical home. *Journal of the American Medical Association*, 300: 834–5.

Barsevick, A. M., Sweeney, C., Haney, E., and Chung, E. (2002). A systematic qualitative analysis of psychoeducational interventions for depression in patients with cancer. *Oncology Nursing Forum*, 29(1): 73–84.

Bateson, G. (1972). *Steps to an Ecology of Mind*. New York: Ballantine.

Baxter, L. A., and Montgomery, B. M. (1996). *Relating: Dialogues and Dialectics*. New York: Guilford.

Beach, M. C., et al. (2004) What do physicians tell patients about themselves? A qualitative analysis of physician self-disclosure. *Journal of General Internal Medicine*, 19: 911–16.

Beck, C. S. (2001). *Communicating for Better Health: A Guide through the Medical Mazes*. Boston, MA: Allyn and Bacon.

Beck, C. S., Ragan, S. L., and du Pré, A. (1997). *Partnership for Health: Building Relationships between Women and Health Caregivers*. Mahwah, NJ: Erlbaum.

Beck, C. S., et al. (2004). Enacting "health communication:" The field of health communication as constructed through publication in scholarly journals. *Health Communication*, 16: 475–92.

Beck, R. S., Daughtridge, R., and Sloan, P. D. (2002). Physician–Patient communication in the primary care office: A systematic review. *Journal of the American Board of Family Practice*, 15: 25–38.

Becker, T., Rogers, E., and Sopory, P. (1992). *Designing Health Communication Campaigns: What Works?* Newbury Park: Sage.

Bedford, V. H., and Blieszner, R. (2000). Personal relationships in later life families. In R. M. Milardo and S. Duck (eds), *Families as Relationships* (pp. 157–74). San Francisco, CA: John Wiley.

Bellet, P. S., and Maloney, M. J. (1991). The importance of empathy as an interviewing skill in medicine. *Journal of the American Medical Association*, 266: 1831–2.

Belluck, P. (2009, November 17). Many doctors to stay course on breast exams for now. *The New York Times*. Available at: <http://www.nytimes.com/2009/11/18/health/18doctors.html?emc=eta1>.

Berger, C. R., and Calabrese, R. J. (1975). Some explorations in initial interaction and beyond: Toward a developmental theory of interpersonal communication. *Human Communication Theory*, 1: 99–112.

Berger, C. R., and Kellerman, K. A. (1983). To ask or not to ask: Is that a question? In R. M. Bostrom (ed.), *Communication Yearbook* (pp. 342–68). Newbury Park, CA: Sage.

Berkman, L. F., and Syme, L. S. (1979). Social networks, host resistance, and mortality: A nine-year follow-up study of Alameda County residents. *Journal of Epidemiology*, 109: 186–204.

Berlo, D. K. (1960). *The Process of Communication*. New York: Holt, Rinehart and Winston, Inc.

Bernabei, R. et al. (1998). Management of pain in elderly patients with cancer. *Journal of the American Medical Association*, 279: 1877–82.

Bernhardt, J. M. (2001). Tailoring messages and design in a web-based skin cancer prevention intervention. *International Electronic Journal of Health Education*, 4: 290–7.

Berry, J. A. (2009). Nurse practitioner/patient communication styles in clinical practice. *Journal of the American Academy of Nurse Practitioners*, 5: 508–15.

Berwick, D. (2002). *Escape Fire*. New York: The Commonwealth Fund.

Bethea (Sparks), L. S., Travis, S. S., and Pecchioni, L. (2000). Family caregivers' use of humor in conveying information about caring for dependent older adults. *Health Communication*, 12: 361–76.

Bevan, J. L. (2009). Interpersonal communication apprehension, topic avoidance, and the experience of Irritable Bowel Syndrome. *Personal Relationships*, 16: 147–65.

Bevan, J. L., Finan, A., and Kaminsky, A. (2008). Modeling serial arguments in close relationships: The serial argument process model. *Human Communication Research*, 34: 600–24.

Bevan, J. and Sparks, L. (2010). Communication in the context of distance caregiving. Paper presented at the International Communication Association, Singapore.

Bierman, J. S., Golladay, G. J., Greenfield, M. L., and Baker, L. H. (1999). Evaluation of cancer information on the internet. *Cancer*, 86: 381–90.

Billings, A. G., and Moos, R. H. (1981). The role of coping responses and social resources in attenuating the impact of stressful life events. *Journal of Behavioral Medicine*, 4: 139–57.

Birdwhistell, R. L. (1970). *Kinesics and Context*. Philadelphia, PA: University of Pennsylvania Press.

Blackhall, L. J., et al. (1995). Ethnicity and attitudes toward patient autonomy. *Journal of the American Medical Association*, 274: 820–5.

Blevins, D., and Deason-Howell (2002). End-of-life care in nursing homes: The interface of policy, research, and practice. *Behavioral Sciences and the Law*, 20: 271–86.

Block, S. D., and Sullivan, A. M. (1998). Attitudes about end-of-life care: A national cross-sectional study. *Journal of Palliative Medicine*, 1: 347–55.

Bloom, J. R. (1982). Social support, accommodation to stress and adjustment to breast cancer. *Social Science Medicine*, 16: 1329–38.

Bloom, J. R., and Spiegel, D. (1984). The relationship of two dimensions of social support to the psychological well-being and social functioning of women with advanced breast cancer. *Social Science Medicine*, 19: 831–7.

Booth-Butterfield, M. (2003). Embedded health behaviors from adolescence to adulthood: The impact of tobacco. *Health Communication*, 15: 171–85.

Bormann, E. G. (1972). Fantasies and rhetorical vision: The rhetorical criticism of social reality, *Quarterly Journal of Speech*, 58: 1972, 396–407.

Bormann, E. G. (1975). *Discussion and Ground Methods,* New York: Harper and Row.

Bormann, E. G. (1977). Fetching good out of evil: A rhetorical use of calamity. *Quarterly Journal of Speech*, 63: 130–9.

Bormann, E. G. (1982). The symbolic convergence theory of communication: Applications and implications for teachers and consultants. *Journal of Applied Communication*, 10: 50–61.

Bourgeois, F., et al. (2008). Evaluation of influenza prevention in the workplace using personally controlled health records: Randomized control trial. *Journal of Medical Internet Research*, 10: e5.

Bourhis, R. Y., and Giles, H. (1977). The language of intergroup distinctiveness. In H. Giles (ed.), *Language, Ethnicity and Intergroup Relations* (pp. 119–35). London: Academic Press.

Bowyer, M. W., et al. (2009). Teaching breaking bad news using mixed reality simulation. *Journal of Surgical Research*, 151(2): 182–3.

Bradac, J. J. (2001). Theory comparison: Uncertainty reduction, problematic integration, uncertainty management, and other curious constructs. *Journal of Communication*, 51: 456–76.

Bradley, C. J. (2005). The need for online information on the economic consequences of cancer diagnosis. *Journal of Medical Internet Research*, 7: e29.

Branscombe, N. R., Schmitt, M. T., and Harvey, R. D. (1999). Perceiving pervasive discrimination among African Americans: Implications for group identification and well-being. *Journal of Personality and Social Psychology*, 77: 135–49.

Brashers, D. E. (2001). Communication and uncertainty management. *Journal of Communication*, 51: 477–97.

Brashers, D. E., Haas, S. M., and Neidig, J. L. (1999). The patient self-advocacy scale: Measuring patient involvement in health care decision making interactions. *Health Communication*, 11: 97–121.

Brashers, D. E., et al. (2000). Communication in the management of uncertainty: The case of persons living with HIV or AIDS. *Communication Monographs*, 67: 63–84.

Brereton, L., and Nolan, M. (2000). 'You do know he's had a stroke, don't you?': Preparation for family caregiving – the neglected dimension. *Journal of Clinical Nursing*, 9: 498–506.

Brescia, F. J., Portenoy, R. K., Ryan, M., Krasnoff, L., and Gray, G. (1992). Pain, opioid use, and survival in hospitalized patients with advanced cancer. *Journal of Clinical Oncology*, 10: 149–55.

Brewer, M. (1979). In-group bias in the minimal intergroup situation: A cognitive–motivational analysis. *Psychological Bulletin*, 86: 307–34.

Brewer, M. B., and Miller, N. (1988). Contact and cooperation: When do they work? In P. A. Katz and D. A. Taylor (eds), *Eliminating Racism* (pp. 315–26). New York: Plenum Press.

Brod, M., and Heurtin-Roberts, S. (1992). Older Russian émigrés and medical care. *The Western Journal of Medicine*, 157: 333–6.

Brogan, C. (2008, August 13). *My Best Advice about Social Networking* [Web log message]. Retrieved from: <http://www.chrisbrogan.com/my-best-advice-about-social-net working/>.

Brogan, C., and Smith, J. (2009). *Trust Agents: Using the Web to Build Influence, Improve Reputation, and Earn Trust*. Hobokken, NJ: Wiley.

Bronfin, (2008). Teaching the art and science of the clinical interview: The pediatrician as mentor. *Clinical Pediatrics*, 47: 531–4.

Brooks, R. G., and Menachemi, N. (2006). Physicians' use of email with patients: Factors influencing electronic communication and adherence to best practices. *Journal of Medical Internet Research*, 8: e2.

Brown, J., Stewart, M., and Ryan, B. L. (2001). *Assessing Communication between Patients and Physicians: The Measure of Patient-centered Communication*. London: Thames Valley Family Practice Research Unit.

Brown, R. F., et al. (2002). Responding to the active and passive patient: Flexibility is the key. *Health Expectations*, 15: 236–45.

Brubaker, R. G., and Wickersham, D. (1990). Encouraging the practice of testicular self-examination: A field application of the theory of reasoned action. *Health Psychology*, 9: 154–63.

Buckman, R. (1996). Talking to patients about cancer. *British Medical Journal*, 31: 699–700.

Buckman, R. (2005). Breaking bad news: The S-P-I-K-E-S strategy. *Community Oncology*, 2 (March/April): 138–42.

Buckman, R., and Baile, W. (2007). Truth telling: Yes, but how? *Journal of Clinical Oncology*, 25: 3181.

Buckman, R., Lipkin, M., Sourkes, B., and Tolle, S. (1997). Strategies and skills for breaking bad news. *Patient Care*, 31(11): 61–71.

Buller, D. B. (1986). Distraction during persuasive communication: A meta-analytic review. *Communication Monographs*, 53(2): 91114.

Burgoon, J. K. (1995). Cross-cultural and intercultural applications of expectancy violations theory. In R. L. Wiseman (ed.), *Intercultural Communication Theory* (pp. 194–214). Thousand Oaks, CA: Sage.

Burgoon, J. K., Stern, L. A., and Dillman, L. (1995). *Interpersonal Adaptation: Dyadic Interaction Patterns*. New York: Cambridge University Press.

Burleson, B. R. (1990). Comforting as social support: Relational consequences of supportive behaviors. In S. Duck and R. C. Silver (eds), *Personal Relationships and Social Support* (pp. 66–82). Newbury Park, CA: Sage.

Burleson, B. R. (1994). Comforting messages: Significance, approaches, and effects. In B. R. Burleson, T. L. Albrecht, and I. G. Sarason (eds), *Communication of Social Support: Messages, Interactions, Relationships and Community* (pp. 3–28). Newbury Park, CA: Sage.

Burleson, B. R. (2003a). Emotional support skill. In J. O. Greene and B. R. Burleson (eds), *Handbook of Communication and Social Interaction Skills* (pp. 551–94). Mahwah, NJ: Erlbaum.

Burleson, B. R. (2003b). The experience and effects of emotional support: What the study of cultural and gender differences can tell us about close relationships, emotion, and interpersonal communication. *Personal Relationships*, 10: 1–23.

Burleson, B. R. (2009). Understanding the outcomes of supportive communication: A dual-process approach. *Journal of Social and Personal Relationships*, 26: 21–38.

Burleson, B. R., and Caplan, S. (forthcoming). Cognitive complexity. In J. C. McCroskey, J. A. Daly, and M. M. Martin (eds), *Communication and Personality: Trait Perspectives*. Cresskill, NJ: Hampton Press.

Butow, P. N., et al. (1996). When the diagnosis is cancer: Patient communication experiences and preferences. *Cancer*, 77: 2630–7.

Bylund, C., and MaKoul, G. (2005). Examining empathy in medical encounters: An observational study using the empathic communication coding system. *Health Communication*, 18: 123–40.

Byock, I. (2000). Completing the continuum of cancer care: Integrating life-prolongation and palliation. *CA: A Cancer Journal for Clinicians*, 50: 123–32.

Cacioppo, J. T., Harkins, S. G., and Petty, R. E. (1981). The nature of attitudes and cognitive responses and their relationship to behavior. In R. E. Petty, T. M. Ostrom, and T. C. Brock (eds), *Cognitive Responses in Persuasion* (pp. 31–54). Hillsdale, N.J.: Erlbaum.

Cacioppo, J. T., and Petty, R. E. (1979). Effects of message reception on argument processing, recall, and persuasion. *Basic and Applied Social Psychology*, 10: 3–12.

Cacioppo, J. T., Petty, R. E., Kao, C. F., and Rodriguez, R. (1986). Central and peripheral routes to persuasion: An individual difference perspective. *Journal of Personality and Social Psychology*, 51: 1032–43.

Callahan, M. (2009, April 7). Tech-savvy patients and pros work up healthcare 2.0. *The New York Post*. Retrieved from: <http://www.nypost.com/p/lifestyle/health/item_K2qlmtJGUaONAh2CeedEiN>.

Canary, D. J., Cody, M. J., and Manusov, V. L. (2000). *Interpersonal Communication: A Goals Based Approach* (2nd ed.). Boston, MA: Bedford/St. Martin's Press.

Canary, D. J., Cupach, W. R., and Serpe, R. T. (2001). A competence-based approach to examining interpersonal conflict: Test of a longitudinal model. *Communication Research*, 28: 79–104.

Cantor, M., and Brennan, M. (2000). *Social Care of the Elderly: The Effects of Ethnicity, Class, and Culture*. New York: Springer.

Carbone, E. T., et al. (2007). Diabetes self-management: Perspectives of Latino patients and their health care providers. *Patient Education and Counseling*, 66: 202–10.

Carstensen, L. L. (1991). Selectivity theory: Social activity in life-span context. *Annual Review of Gerontology and Geriatrics*, 11: 195–217.

Carstensen, L. L. (1992). Social and emotional patterns in adulthood: Support for socioe-motional selectivity theory. *Psychology and Aging*, 7: 331–8.

Cass, A., et al. (2002). Sharing the true stories: Improving communication between Aboriginal patients and healthcare workers. *Medical Journal of Australia*, 176: 466–70.

Caughlin, J. P., and Afifi, T. A. (2004). When is topic avoidance unsatisfying? Examining moderators of the association between avoidance and dissatisfaction. *Human Communication Research*, 30: 479–513.

Cawyer, C., and Smith-duPré, A. (1995). Communicating social support: Identifying supportive episodes in an HIV/AIDS support group. *Communication Quarterly*, 43: 243–58.

Cegala, D. J., McClure, L., Marinelli, T. M., and Post, D. M. (2000). The effects of communication skills training on patients' participation during medical interviews. *Patient Education and Counseling*, 41: 209–22.

Centers for Disease Control and Prevention (2004). *Vital and Health Statistics*. Retrieved from: <http://www.cdc.gov/>.

Centers for Disease Control and Prevention (2009). *Sexually Transmitted Diseases Surveillance, 2008*. Retrieved from: <http://www.cdc.gov/std/stats08/main.htm>.

Chaiken, S. (1980). Heuristic versus systematic information processing and the use of source versus message cues in persuasion. *Journal of Personality and Social Psychology*, 39: 752–66.

Chakrabarty, A., and Geisse, J. K. (2004). Medical therapies for non-melanoma skin cancer. *Clinics in Dermatology*, 22: 183–8.

Chang, A., and Bordia, P. (2001). A multidisciplinary approach to group cohesion–group performance relationship. *Small Group Research*, 32: 379–405.

Charles, C. A., Gafni, A., Whelan, T., and O'Brien, M. A. (2005). Treatment decision aids: Conceptual issues and future directions. *Health Expectations*, 8: 114–25.

Charmaz, K. (1999). From the "sick role" to stories of self: Understanding the self in illness. In R. J. Contrada and R. D. Ashmore (eds), *Self, Social Identity, and Physical Health: Interdisciplinary Explorations* (pp. 209–39). New York: Oxford University Press.

Chen, G. M., and Starosta, W. J. (1998). *Foundations of Intercultural Communication*. Boston, MA: Allyn and Bacon.

Chen, X., and Silverstein, M. (2000). Intergenerational social support and the psychological well-being of older parents in China. *Research on Aging*, 22: 43–65.

Cheney, G. (1983). On the various and changing meanings of organizational membership: A field study of organizational identification. *Communication Monographs*, 50: 342–62.

Cheng, C., and Pickler, R. H. (2009). Effects of stress and social support on postpartum health of Chinese mothers in the United States. *Research in Nursing and Health*, 32: 582–91.

Chesler, M. A., and Barbarin, O. A. (1984). Difficulties of providing help in a crisis: Relationships between parents of children with cancer and their friends. *Journal of Social Issues*, 40: 113–34.

Chew, F., Palmer, S., and Kim, S. (1998). Testing the influence of the health belief model and a television program on nutrition behavior. *Health Communication*, 10: 227–45.

Christakis, N. A., and Fowler, J. H. (2009). *Connected: The Surprising Power of Our Social Networks and How They Shape Our Lives.* New York: Little, Brown and Company.

Clark, N. M., et al. (2009). Consideration of shared decision making in nursing: A review of clinicians' perceptions and interventions. *Open Nursing Journal*, 3: 65–75.

Clarke, G., et al. (2002). Overcoming depression on the Internet (ODIN): A randomized controlled trial of an Internet depression skills intervention program. *Journal of Medical Internet Research*, 4: e14.

Clarke, L. (1995). Family care and changing family structure: Bad news for the elderly? In I. Allen and E. Perkins (eds), *The Future of Family Care for Older People* (pp. 19–49). London: HMSO.

Cline, R. J. (1999). Communication within social support groups. In L. R. Frey (ed.), D. S. Gouran, and M. S. Poole (assoc. eds), *The Handbook of Group Communication Theory and Research* (pp. 516–38). Thousand Oaks, CA: Sage.

Cluck, G. G., and Cline, R. W. (1989). The circle of others: Self-help groups for the bereaved. *Communication Quarterly*, 34: 306–25.

Cohen, S. (1988). Psychosocial models of the role of support in the etiology of physical disease. *Health Psychology*, 7: 269–97.

Cohen, S., and Wills, T. A. (1985). Stress, social support, and the buffering hypothesis. *Psychological Bulletin*, 98: 310–57.

Cole, S. W., Kemeny, M. E., Taylor, S. E., and Visscher, B. R. (1996). Elevated physical health risk among gay men who conceal their homosexual identity. *Health Psychology*, 15 (4): 243–51.

Collins, D., Villagran, M. M., and Sparks, L. (2008). Crossing borders, crossing cultures: Barriers to cancer prevention and treatment along the U.S./Mexico border. *Patient Education and Counseling*, 71(3): 333–9.

Committee on Health Literacy, Institute of Medicine (2004). Nielsen-Bohlman, L. N., Panzer, A. M., Kindig, D. A. (eds) *Health Literacy: A Prescription to End Confusion.* Washington, DC: The National Academies Press.

The Commonwealth Fund (2009). Do primary care physicians treating minority patients report problems delivering high–quality care? charts. Retrieved from: <http://www.commonwealthfund.org/Charts-and-Maps/ChartCart/View-All.aspx?chartcategory=Do+Primary+Care+Physicians+Treating+Minority+Patients+Report+Problems+Delivering+High+Quality+Care>.

Connidis, I. A., and Kemp, C. L. (2008). Negotiating actual and anticipated parental support: Multiple sibling voices in three-generation families. *Journal of Aging Studies*, 22: 229–38.

Connor, S. R., et al. (2002). Interdisciplinary approaches to assisting with end-of-life care and decision making. *American Behavioral Scientist*, 46: 340–56.

Conrad, P. (1987). The experience of illness: Recent and new directions. In J. Roth and P. Conrad (eds), *Research in the Sociology of Health Care: A Research Manual* (Vol. 6, pp. 1–31). Greenwich, CT: JAL.

Contrada, R. J. (1989). Type A behavior, personality hardiness, and cardiovascular responses to stress. *Journal of Personality & Social Psychology*, 57: 895–903.

Contrada, R. J., and Ashmore, R. D. (1999a). Introduction: Self and social identity: Key to understanding social and behavioral aspects of physical health and disease? In R. J. Contrada and R. D. Ashmore (eds), *Self, Social Identity, and Physical Health: Interdisciplinary Explorations* (pp. 3–21). New York: Oxford University Press.

Contrada and R. D. Ashmore (eds). (1999b). *Self, Social Identity, and Physical Health: Interdisciplinary Explorations* (pp. 209–39). New York: Oxford University Press.

Cooney, E. (2010, January 11). Looking at final options. *The Boston Globe.* Retrieved from: <http://www.boston.com/news/health/articles/2010/01/11/ angelo_volandes_gives_patients_a_look_at_all_their_end_of_life_options/>.

Cooper, L. A., et al. (2003). Patient-centered communication, ratings of care, and concordance of patient and physician race. *Annals of Internal Medicine*, 139: 907–15.

Cooper, P. (1995). *Communication for the Classroom Teacher* (5th edn). Scottsdale, AZ: Gorsuch Scarisbrick.

Coopman, S. J. (2001). Democracy, performance, and outcomes in interdisciplinary health care teams. *The Journal of Business Communication*, 38: 261–84.

Cora-Bramble, D., and Williams, L. (2000). Explaining illness to Latinos: Cultural foundations and messages. In Whaley, B. B. (ed.), *Explaining Illness: Research, Theory, and Structure* (pp. 259–79). Mahwah, NJ: Erlbaum.

Corr, C. A., Nabe, C. M., and Corr, D. M. (1997) *Death and Dying, Life and Living* (2nd edn). Pacific Grove, CA: Brooks/Cole Publishing Company.

Coupland, J. (2003). Ageist ideology and discourses of control in skin care product advertising. In J. Coupland and R. Gwyn (eds), *Discourse, Identity and the Body* (pp. 127–50). London: Palgrave.

Coupland, N. (2004). Age in social and sociolinguistic theory, In J. F. Nussbaum and J. Coupland (eds), *Handbook of Communication and Aging Research* (pp. 69–91). Mahwah, NJ: Erlbaum.

Coupland, N., Coupland, J., Giles, H., and Henwood, K. (1988). Accommodating the elderly: Invoking and extending the theory. *Language in Society*, 17: 1–41.

Coupland, N., Coupland, J., and Giles, H. (1991). Telling age in later life: Identity and face implications. *Text*, 9: 129–51.

Coyne, C. A., et al. (2003). Randomized, controlled trial of an easy-to-read informed consent statement for clinical trial participation: A study of the Eastern Cooperative Oncology Group. *Journal of Clinical Oncology*, 21: 836–42.

Cragan, J. F. (1975). Rhetorical strategy: A dramatist interpretation and application. *Central States Speech Journal*, 26: 4–11.

Cragan, J., and Shields, D. C. (1977). Foreign policy communication dramas: How mediated rhetoric played in the Peoria campaign 176. *Quarterly Journal of Speech*, 63: 274–89.

Crane, K. M. (2005, November 10). Telemedicine's remote control; virtual health exams cut costs of treating an aging population. *Wall Street Journal* [Eastern edition]: B8.

Crawford, T. J., and Boyer, R. (1985). Salient consequences, cultural values, and childbearing intentions. *Journal of Applied Social Psychology*, 15: 16–30.

Creagan, E. T. (1997). Attitude and disposition: Do they make a difference in cancer survival? *Mayo Clinic Proceedings*, 72 (2): 160–4.

Crocker, J., and Major, B. (1989). Social stigma and self-esteem: The self–protective properties of stigma. *Psychological Review*, 96: 608–30.

Crockett, W. H. (1965). Cognitive complexity and impression formation. In B. A. Maher (ed.), *Progress in Experimental Personality Research* (Vol. 2, pp. 47–90). New York: Academic Press.

Cummins, C. O., et al. (2003). Development of research criteria to evaluate health behavior change websites. *Journal of Health Psychology*, 8: 55–62.

Cwikel, J. M., and Isreal, B. A. (1987). Examining mechanisms of social support and social networks: A review of health-related intervention studies. *Public Health Review*, 15: 159–93.

Czaja, R., Manfredi, C., and Price, J. (2003). The determinants and consequences of information seeking among cancer patients. *Journal of Health Communication*, 8: 529–62.

Dakof, G. A., and Taylor, S. E. (1990). Victim's perceptions of social support: What is helpful from whom? *Journal of Personality and Social Psychology*, 58: 80–9.

Davidhizar, R. (1999). Caregiving from a distance. *Hospital Topics*, 77: 9–13.

Davis, T.C., et al. (2001). The role of inadequate health literacy skills in colorectal cancer screening. *Cancer Investigation*, 19: 193–200.

Davis, T. C., et al. (2002). Health literacy and cancer communication. *CA: A Cancer Journal for Clinicians*, 52(3): 134–54.

Davis, T. C. et al. (2006). Literacy and misunderstanding prescription drug labels. *Annals of Internal Medicine*, 145: 887–95.

Davison, K. P., Pennebaker, J. W., and Dickerson, S. S. (2000). Who talks? The social psychology of illness support groups. *American Psychologist*, 55: 205–17.

Dean, A., and Lin, N. (1977). The stress buffering role of social support: Problems and prospects for systematic investigation. *Journal of Health and Social Behavior*, 32: 321–41.

Dean, K. (1989). Self-care components of lifestyles. *Social Science and Medicine*, 29: 137–52.

Dean, K. (1996). Using theory to guide policy relevant health promotion research. *Health Promotion International*, 11: 19–26.

Dee, C. R., Teolis, M., and Todd, A. D. (2005). Physicians' use of the personal digital assistant (PDA) in clinical decision-making. *Journal of the Medical Library Association*, 93: 480–6.

Deimling, G., Kahana, B., and Schumacher, J. (1997). Life threatening illness: The transition from victim to survivor. *Journal of Aging and Identity*, 2: 165–86.

Delgado, M. (1998). *Latino Elders and the Twenty-first Century: Issues and Challenges for Culturally Competent Research and Practice*. Binghamton, NY: Haworth Press.

Demiris, G., et al. (2008). Use of videophones for distance caregiving: An enriching experience for families and residents in long-term care. *Journal of Gerontological Nursing*, 7: 50–5.

DeWalt, D. A., and Pignone, M. P. (2005a). Reading is fundamental: The relationship between literacy and health. *Archives of Internal Medicine*, 165: 1943–5.

DeWalt, D. A., and Pignone, M. P. (2005b). The role of literacy in health and health care. *American Family Physician*, 72: 387.

De Wit, D. J., Wister, A. V., and Burch, T. K. (1988). Physical distance and social contact between elders and their adult children. *Research on Aging*, 10: 56–80.

Dibbelt, S., Schaidhammer, M., Fleischer, C., and Greitemann, B. (2009). Patient–doctor interaction in rehabilitation: The relationship between perceived interaction quality and long-term treatment results. *Patient Education and Counseling*, 76: 328–35.

DiClemente, C. C., and Prochaska, J. O. (1985). Processes and stages of change: Coping and competence in smoking behavior change. In S. Shiffman and T. A. Willis (eds), *Coping and Substance Abuse* (pp. 319–34). San Diego, CA: Academic Press.

Dillow, M. R., Neary Dunleavy, K., and Weber, K. D. (2009). The impact of relational characteristics and reasons for topic avoidance on relational closeness. *Communication Quarterly*, 57(2): 205–23.

DiMatteo, M., and Hays, R. (1981). Social support and serious illness. In B. Gottlieb (ed.), *Social Networks and Social Support* (pp. 117–48). Beverly Hills, CA: Sage.

Dion, K. L., Dion, K. K., and Pak, A. W. (1992). Personality-based hardiness as a buffer for discrimination-related stress in members of Toronto's Chinese community. *Canadian Journal of Behavioral Science*, 24: 517–36.

Dolin, D. J., and Booth-Butterfield, S. (1995). Foot-in-the-door and cancer prevention. *Health Communication*, 7: 55–64.

Donnelly, S., Walsh, D., and Rybicki, L. (1994). The symptoms of advanced cancer in 1,000 patients. *Journal of Palliative Care*, 10: 57.

Donohew, L., and Ray, E. B. (eds). (1990). *Communication and Health*. Hillsdale, NJ: Lawrence Erlbaum.

Dracup, K., et al. (1994). Counseling, education, and lifestyle modifications. *Journal of the American Medical Association*, 263: 1816–19.

Dreyer, E. A. (1994). *Earth Crammed with Heaven: A Spirituality of Everyday Life.* Mahwah, New Jersey: Paulist Press.

Dryden, C., and Giles, H. (1987). Language, social identity, and health. In H. Beloff and A. M. Coleman (eds), *Psychology survey* (pp. 115–138). Leicester: British Psychological Society.

Duggan, A. P., and Bradshaw, Y. S. (2008). Mutual influence processes in physician-patient communication: An interaction adaptation perspective. *Communication Research Reports,* 25(3): 211–26.

Dunkel-Schetter, C., and Bennett, T. L. (1990). Differentiating the cognitive and behavioral aspects of social support. In I. G. Sarason, B. R. Sarason, and G. R. Pierce (eds), *Social Support: An Interactional View* (pp. 267–96). New York: Wiley.

du Pré, A. (1998). *Humor and the Healing Arts: Multimethod Analysis of Humor Use in Health Care.* Mahwah, NJ: Lawrence Erlbaum Associates.

du Pré, A. (2001). *Communicating about Health: Current Issues and Perspectives.* Mountain View, CA: Mayfield.

du Pré, A. (2002). Accomplishing the impossible: Talking about body *and* mind *and* soul during a medical visit. *Health Communication,* 14: 1–21.

du Pré, A. (2005a). *Communicating about Health: Current Issues and Perspectives* (2nd edn). New York: McGraw-Hill.

du Pré, A. (2005b). Making empowerment work: Medical center soars in satisfaction ratings. In E. B. Ray (ed.), *Case Studies in Health Communication.* Mahwah, NJ: Erlbaum Associates.

du Pré, A., and Beck, C. (1997). "How can I put this?" Exaggerated self-disparagement as alignment strategy during problematic disclosures by patients to doctors. *Qualitative Health Research,* 7(4): 487–503.

du Pré, A., and Lepper, T. S. (forthcoming). Meridians and mind-body congruence: Spiritual aspects of healing in a homeopathic care setting. In M. Wills (ed.), *Communicating Spirituality in Health Care.* Cresskill, NJ: Hampton.

du Pré, A., and Ray, E. B. (2008). Comforting episodes: Transcendent experiences of cancer survivors. In L. Sparks, D. O'Hair, and G. L. Kreps (eds), *Cancer Communication and Aging* (pp. 99–114). Cresskill, NJ: Hampton.

Dutta, M. (2008). Communicating health: A culture-centered approach. Cambridge: Polity.

Dutta-Bergman, M. (2004). The unheard voices of Santalis: Communicating about health from the margins of India. *Communication Theory,* 14: 237–263.

Eagle, L. C., Hawkins, J. C., Styles, E., and Reid, J. (2006) Breaking through the invisible barrier of low functional literacy: Implications for health communication. *Studies in Community Science,* 5(2): 29–55.

Eagly, A. H., and Chaiken, S. (1993). *The Psychology of Attitudes.* Fort Worth: Harcourt Bruce Jovanovich College Publishers.

Eckes, T. (1994). Explorations in gender cognition: Content and structure of female and male subtypes. *Social Cognition,* 12: 37–60.

Edwards, C. C., and Harwood, J. (2003). Social identity in the classroom: An examination of age identification between students and instructors. *Communication Education,* 52: 60–5.

Edwards, H., and Noller, P. (1998). Factors influencing caregiver–care receiver communication and the impact on the well-being of older care receivers. *Health Communication,* 10: 317–42.

Edwards, J. M., and Trimble, K. (1992). Anxiety, coping, and academic performance. *Anxiety, Stress, and Coping,* 5: 337–50.

Egbert, N., Mickley, J., and Coeling, H. (2004). A review and application of social scientific measures of religiosity and spirituality: Assessing a missing component in health communication research. *Health Communication,* 16: 7–27.

Egbert, N., and Parrott, R. (2003). Empathy and social support for the terminally ill: Implications for recruiting and retaining hospice and hospital volunteers. *Communication Studies*, 54: 18–34.

Egbert, N., Sparks, L., Kreps, G. L., and du Pré, A. (2008). Finding meaning in the journey: Methods of spiritual coping for aging cancer patients. In L. Sparks, H. D. O'Hair, and G. L. Kreps, (eds), *Cancer Communication and Aging* (pp. 277–92). Cresskill, NJ: Hampton Press.

Eggly, S. (2002) Physician–patient co-construction of illness narratives in the medical interview. *Health Communication* 14: 339–60.

Eisen, M., Zellman, G. I., and McAllister, A. L. (1985). A health belief model approach to adolescents' fertility control: Some pilot program findings. *Health Education Quarterly*, 12: 185–210.

Eldh, A. C., Ekman, I., and Ehnfors, M. (2006). Conditions for patient participation and non-participation in health care. *Nursing Ethics*, 13: 503–14.

Elliot, B. A., et al. (1996). Patients and family members: The role of knowledge and attitudes in cancer pain. *Journal of Pain and Symptom Management*, 12: 209–20.

Ellingson, L. L. and Buzzanell, P. M. (1999). Listening to women's narratives of breast cancer treatment: A feminist approach to patient satisfaction with physician/patient communication. *Health Communication*, 11: 153–83.

Emanuel, E. J., and Emanuel, L. L. (1992). Four models of the physician patient relationship. *Journal of the American Medical Association*, 267: 2221–6.

Emanuel, E. J., and Emanuel, L. L. (1998). The promise of a good death. *Lancet*, 351: 21–9.

Endler, N. S., and Parker, J. D. A. (1990). Multidimensional assessment of coping: A critical evaluation. *Journal of Personality and Social Psychology*, 58: 844–54.

Eng, T. R. (2001). *The e-Health Landscape: A Terrain Map of Emerging Information and Communication Technologies in Health and Healthcare*. Princeton, NJ: The Robert Wood Johnson Foundation.

Epstein, R. and Street, R. (2007). *Patient-centered Communication in Cancer Care: Promoting Healing, and Reducing Suffering* (NCI Publication No. 07-6225).

Epstein, R. M., Alper, B. S., and Quill, T. E. (2004). Communicating evidence for participatory decision making. *Journal of the American Medical Association*, 291: 2359–66.

Epstein, R. M., et al. (2007). Exploring and validating patient concerns: Relation to prescribing for depression. *Annals of Family Medicine*, 5: 21–8.

Evans, W. G., Tulsky, J. A., Back, A. L., and Arnold, R. M. (2006). Communication at times of transitions: How to help patients cope with loss and re-define hope. *The Cancer Journal*, 12: 417–24.

Eysenck, H. J. (1994). Cancer, personality and stress: Prediction and prevention. *Advances in Behaviour Research and Therapy*, 16(3): 167–215.

Eysenck, H. J. (1995). The causal role of stress and personality in the aetiology of cancer and coronary heart disease. In C. D. Spielberger and I. G. Sarason (eds), *Stress and Emotion: Anxiety, Anger and Curiosity* (pp. 3–12). Philadelphia, PA: Taylor and Francis.

Facione, N. C. (2002). Perceived risk of breast cancer. *Cancer*, 10: 256–261.

Falomir, J. M., and Invernizzi, F. (1999). The role of social influence and smoker identity in resistance to smoking cessation. *Swiss Journal of Psychology*, 58(2): 73–84.

Farrell M. J., and Rose L. (2008). Use of mobile handheld computers in clinical nursing education. *Journal of Nursing Education*, 47: 13–19.

Ferguson, K. J., Yesalis, C. E., Pomrehn, P. R., and Kirkpatrick, M. B. (1989). Attitudes, knowledge, and beliefs as predictors of exercise intent and behavior in schoolchildren. *Journal of School Health*, 59: 112–15.

Ferguson, T. (1998). Digital-doctoring: Opportunities and challenges in electronic patient–physician communication. *Journal of the American Medical Association*, 280: 1361–2.

Fernar, R. E., and Aronson, J. K. (2000). Medication errors, worse than a crime. *The Lancet*, 355: 947–8.

Ferraro, K. F. (2004). Next steps in understanding the prayer/health connection. In K. W. Schaie, N. Krause, and A. Booth (eds), *Religious Influences on Health and Well-being in the Elderly* (pp. 96–103). New York: Springer.

Ferraro, K. F. (2005). Health and aging. In R. H. Binstock, and L. K. George, S. Cutler, J. Hendricks, and J. Schulz (eds), *Handbook of Aging and the Social Sciences* (6th edn). Burlington, MA: Elsevier.

Festinger, L. (1954). A theory of social comparison processes. *Human Relations*, 2: 117–40.

Festinger, L., and Maccoby, N. (1964). On resistance to persuasive communications. *Journal of Abnormal Psychology*, 68: 359–66.

Field, M. J., and Cassel, C. K. (eds). (1997). *Approaching Death: Improving Care at the End of Life*. Washington, DC: National Academy Press.

Fields, D., and Howells, K. (1985). Medical students' self-reported worries about aspects of death and dying. *Death Studies*, 10: 147–54.

Finch, J., and Mason, J. (1993). *Negotiating Family Responsibilities*. London: Tavistock/ Routledge.

Firth-Cozens, J. (1993). Stress, psychological problems and clinical performance. In C. Vincent, M. Ennis, and R. J. Audley (eds), *Medical Accidents*. Oxford: Oxford University Press.

Fiscella, K., Franks, P., Gold, M. R., and Clancy, C. M. (2000). Inequality in quality: Addressing socioeconomic, racial and ethnic disparities in health care. *The Journal of the American Medical Association*, 283: 2579–84.

Fischhoff, B. (1999). Why (cancer) risk communication can be hard. *Journal of the National Cancer Institute Monographs*, 25: 7–13.

Fishbein, M., and Ajzen, I. (1975). *Belief, Attitude, Intention, and Behavior: An Introduction to Theory and Research*. Reading, MA: Addison-Wesley.

Fishbein, M., and Ajzen, I. (1981). Acceptance, yielding and impact: Cognitive processes in persuasion. In R. E. Petty, T. M. Ostrom, and T. C. Brock (eds), *Cognitive Responses in Persuasion* (pp. 339–59). Hillsdale, NJ: Erlbaum.

Fishbein, M., and Middlestadt, S. E. (1989). Using the theory of reasoned action as a framework for understanding and changing AIDS-related behaviors. In V. M. Mays, G. W. Albee, and S. S. Schneider (eds), *Primary Prevention of AIDS: Psychological Approaches* (pp. 93–110). Newbury Park, CA: Sage.

Fishbein, M., Ajzen, I., and McArdle, J. (1980). Changing the behavior of alcoholics: Effects of persuasive communication. In I. Ajzen and M. Fishbein (eds), *Understanding Attitudes and Predicting Social Behavior* (pp. 217–42). Englewood Cliffs, NJ: Prentice-Hall.

Fishbein, M., Middlestadt, S. E., and Hitchcock, P. J. (1991). Using information to change sexually transmitted disease related behaviors: An analysis based on the theory of reasoned action. In J. N. Wasserheit, S. O. Aral, and K. K. Holmes (eds), *Research Issues in Human Behavior Change and Sexually Transmitted Diseases in the AIDS Era* (pp. 243–57). Washington, DC: American Society for Microbiology.

Fisher, J. D., and Fisher, W. A. (2002). The information–motivation–behavioral skills model. In R. J. DiClemente, R. A. Crosby, and M. C. Kegler (eds), *Emerging Theories in Health Promotion Practice and Research: Strategies for Improving Public Health* (pp. 40–70). San Francisco: Josey-Bass.

Fitzpatrick, M. A., and Vangelisti, A. (2001). Communication, relationships, and health. In W. P. Robinson and H. Giles (eds), *The New Handbook of Language and Social Psychology* (pp. 505–30). Chichester, England: Wiley.

Flores, G. (2005). Language barriers to health care in the United States. *New England Journal of Medicine*, 355: 229–31.

Foley, K. M., and Gelband, H. (eds). (2001). *Improving Palliative Care for Cancer.* Washington, DC: National Academy Press.

Folkman, S. and Lazarus, R. S. (1987). Transactional theory and research on emotions and coping. *European Journal of Personality,* 1: 141–69.

Folkman, S., Lazarus, R. S., Pimley, S., and Novacek, J. (1987). Age differences in stress and coping process. *Psychology and Aging,* 2: 171–84.

Ford, S., Fallowfield, L., and Lewis, S. (1996). Doctor–patient interactions in oncology. *Social Science and Medicine,* 42(11): 1511–19.

Ford, T. and Tartaglia, A. (2006). The development, status, and future of healthcare chaplaincy. *Southern Medical Journal,* 99(6): 675–9.

Fowler, C., and Fisher, C. L. (2007, November). *The Effects of Autonomy, Paternalism, and Attitudes about Aging on Parent–Child Discussions of Caregiving.* Paper presented at the annual meeting of the National Communication Association, Chicago, IL.

Fox, S., and Rainie, L. (2000). *The Online Health Care Revolution: How the Web helps Americans Take Better Care of Themselves.* Pew Internet and American Life Project: Online Report. Retrieved from: <http://www.pewinternet.org/reports/pdfs/PIP_Health_Report.pdf>.

Frank, J. D., and Frank, J. B. (1991). *Persuasion and Healing.* Baltimore, MD: John Hopkins University Press.

Frankel, R. (1990). Talking in interviews: A dispreference for patient initiated questions in physician–patient encounters. In G. Psathas (ed.), *Interaction Competence* (pp. 231–62). Lanham, MD: University Press of America.

Franklin, V., et al. (2008). Patients' engagement with "Sweet Talk" – A text messaging support system for young people with diabetes. *Journal of Medical Internet Research,* 10: e20.

Freund, P. E. S., and McGuire, M. (1999). *Health, Illness, and the Social Body: A Critical Sociology.* Upper Saddle River, NJ: Prentice-Hall.

Fritz, G. K., Williams, J. R., and Amylon, M. (1988). After treatment ends: Psychosocial sequelae in pediatric cancer survivors. *American Journal of Orthopsychiatry,* 54: 552–61.

Fryer, D. (1998). Agency restriction. In N. Nicholson (ed.), *The Blackwell Encyclopedia Dictionary of Organizational Behavior* (p. 12). Malden, MA: Blackwell.

Furchtgott-Roth, D. (2009, August 6). Reduce the high cost of medical malpractice. *Reuters.* Retrieved from: <http://blogs.reuters.com/great-debate/2009/08/06/reduce-the-high-cost-of-medical-malpractice/>.

Gany, F., et al. (2007). Patient satisfaction with different interpreting methods: A randomized controlled trial. *Journal of General Internal Medicine,* 22: 312–14.

Garcia, R. (2003, May 9). The misuse of race in medical diagnosis. *The Chronicle of Higher Education,* 49: B15.

Garstka, T. A., Branscombe, N. R., and Hummert, M. L. (2001). *Age group identification in young, middle-aged, and older adults.* Unpublished Manuscript, Gerontology Center, University of Kansas.

Gascoigne, P., Mason, M. D., and Roberts, E. (1999). Factors affecting presentation and delay in patients with testicular cancer: Results of a qualitative study. *Psycho-Oncology,* 8(2): 144–54.

Gazmararian, J., et al. (1999). Health literacy among medicare enrollees in a managed care organization. *Journal of the American Medical Association,* 281(6): 545–51.

Geist-Martin, P., Ray, E. B., and Sharf, B. F. (2003). *Communicating Health: Personal, Cultural, and Political Complexities.* Belmont, CA: Wadsworth/Thomson Learning.

Geist-Martin, P., Sharf, B. F., and Jeha, N. (2008). Communicating health holistically. In H. Zoller and M. Dutta (eds), *Emerging Perspectives in Health Communication: Meaning, Culture, and Power* (pp. 83–112). New York: Routledge.

Gibbs, R. W., and Franks, H. (2002). Embodied metaphor in women's narratives about their experiences with cancer. *Health Communication,* 14(2): 139–65.

Giddens, A. (1984). *The Constitution of Society: Outline of the Theory of Structuration.* Cambridge: Polity.

Gielen, A. C., and McDonald, E. M. (2002). Using the precede–proceed planning model to apply health behavior theories. In K. Glanz, B. K. Rimer, and F. M. Lewis (eds), *Health Behavior and Health Education: Theory, Research, and Practice* (3rd edn, pp. 409–36). San Francisco, CA: Josey-Bass.

Giles, H., Dailey, R. M., Sarkar, J. M., and Makoni, S. (2007). Intergenerational communication beliefs across the lifespan: Comparative data from India. *Communication Reports*, 20: 75–89.

Gillotti, C. M., and Applegate, J. L. (2000). Explaining illness as bad news: Individual differences in explaining illness-related information. In B. B. Whaley (ed.), *Explaining illness: Research, Theory, and Strategies* (pp. 101–20). Mahwah, NJ: Lawrence Erlbaum.

Gillotti, C., Thompson, T., and McNeilis, K. (2002). Communicative competence in the delivery of bad news. *Social Science and Medicine*, 54: 1011–23.

Given, B. A., et al. (1997). Determinants of family caregiver reaction. New and recurrent cancer. *Cancer Practice*, 5: 17–24.

Gloth, F. M. (1998). Foreword. *Hospice Care: A Physician's Guide*. Alexandria, VA National Hospice Organization.

Goffman, E. (1963). *Stigma: Notes on the Management of Spoiled Identity*. Englewood Cliffs, NJ: Prentice-Hall.

Goldsmith, D. J. (2004). *Communicating Social Support*. Cambridge University Press, Cambridge, UK.

Goldsmith, D. J., and Fitch, K. (1997). The normative context of advice as social support. *Human Communication Research*, 23: 454–76.

Goldsmith, J., Wittenberg-Lyles, E., Rodriguez, D., and Sanchez-Reilly, S. (2010). Interdisciplinary geriatric and palliative care team narratives: Collaboration practices and barriers. *Qualitative Health Research*, 20: 93–104.

Google. (2010). *Explore Flu Trends around the World*. Google.org. Retrieved from: <http://www.google.org/flutrends/>.

Gotay, C. C. (2001). Perceptions of informed consent by participants in a prostate cancer prevention study. *Cancer Epidemiology, Biomarkers & Prevention*, 10: 1097–9.

Gouldner, A. W. (1960). The norm of reciprocity: A preliminary statement. *American Sociological Review*, 25(2): 161–78.

Grainger, K. (1995). Communication and the institutionalized elderly. In J. F. Nussbaum and J. Coupland (eds), *Handbook of Communication and Aging Research* (pp. 417–36). Mahwah, NJ: Lawrence Erlbaum Associates.

Grande, G. E., McKerral, A., and Todd, C. J. (2002). Which cancer patients are referred to Hospital at Home for palliative care? *Palliative Medicine*, 16: 115–23.

Granovetter, M. S. (1973). The strength of weak ties. *American Journal of Sociology*, 78: 1360–80.

Graugaard, P. K., Holgersen, K., Eide, H., and Finset, A. (2005). Changes in physician–patient communication from initial to return visits: A prospective study in a hematology outpatient clinic. *Patient Education and Counseling*, 57: 22–9.

Green, L. W., and Kreuter, M. W. (1999). *Health Promotion Planning: An Educational and Environmental Approach* (2nd edn). Mountain View, CA: Mayfield.

Green, L. W., Kreuter, M. W., Deeds, S. G., and Partridge, K. B. (1980). *Health Education Planning: A Diagnostic Approach*. Mountain View, CA: Mayfield.

Greenberg, J., Solomon, S., and Pyszczynski, T. (1997). Terror management theory of self-esteem and cultural worldviews: Empirical assessments and conceptual refinements. In M. Zanna (ed.), *Advances in Experimental Social Psychology* (pp. 61–139). Orlando, FL: Academic Press.

Greene, M. G., and Adelman, R. D. (2001). Building the physician–older patient relationship. In M. L. Hummert and J. F. Nussbaum (eds), *Aging, Communication, and Health:*

Linking Research and Practice for Successful Aging (pp. 101–20). Mahwah, NJ: Lawrence Erlbaum.

Gregg, J. L., and Whitten, P. (2003). *Telehospice: Supporting the Well-being of Caregivers in Rural Areas*. Paper presented at the annual meeting of the International Communication Association, San Diego, CA.

Griffin, R. J., Neuwirth, K., and Dunwoody, S. (1995). Using the theory of reasoned action to examine the health impact of risk messages. *Communication Yearbook*, 18: 201–28.

Grimley, D. M., Riley, G. E., Bellis, J. M., and Prochaska, J. O. (1993). Assessing the stages of change and decision-making for contraceptive use for the prevention of pregnancy, sexually transmitted diseases, and acquired immunodeficiency syndrome. *Health Education Quarterly*, 20: 455–70.

Groopman, J. (2007). *How Doctors Think*. New York: Houghton Mifflin Co.

Grossarth, M. R., et al. (2000). Interaction of psychosocial and physical risk factors in the causation of mammary cancer and its prevention through psychological methods of treatment. *Journal of Clinical Psychology*, 56: 33–50.

Grundy, E. (1995). Demographic influences on the future of family care. In I. Allen and E. Perkins (eds), *The Future of Family Care for Older People* (pp. 1–17). London: HMSO.

Gudykunst, W. B. (1995). Anxiety/uncertainty management (AUM) theory: Current status. In R. L. Wiseman (ed.), *Intercultural Communication Theory* (pp. 8–59). Thousand Oaks, CA: Sage.

Gudykunst, W. B. (1998). *Bridging Differences: Effective Intergroup Communication* (3rd edn). Thousand Oaks, CA: Sage.

Guerrero, L. K., and Afifi, W. A. (1995). What parents don't know: Taboo topics and topic avoidance in parent–child relationships. In T. J. Socha and G. Stamp (eds), *Parents, Children, and Communication: Frontiers of Theory and Research* (pp. 219–45). Hillsdale, NJ: Erlbaum.

Ha, J. (2009). The effects of positive and negative support from children on widowed older adults' psychological adjustment: A longitudinal analysis. *The Gerontologist*. Retrieved from: <http://gerontologist.oxfordjournals.org/cgi/content/short/gnp163v1?rss=1>.

Hahn, S. R. (2009). Patient-centered communication to assess and enhance patient adherence to glaucoma medication. *Ophthalmology*, 116(11): S37–S42.

Haider, M., and Kreps, G. L. (2004). Forty years of diffusion of innovations: Utility and value in public health. *Journal of Health Communication*, 9: 3–12.

Hajek, C., Villagran, M. M., and Wittenberg-Lyles, E. M. (2007). The relationships among perceived physician accommodation, perceived outgroup typicality, and patient inclinations toward compliance. *Communication Research Reports*, 24: 293–302.

Hall, J. A., Horgan, T. G., Stein, T. S., and Roter, D. L. (2002). Liking in the physician-patient relationship. *Patient Education and Counseling*, 48: 69–77.

Hamel, M. B., et al. (2000). Age-related differences in care preferences, treatment decisions, and clinical outcomes of seriously ill hospitalized adults: Lessons from SUPPORT. *Journal of the American Geriatrics Society*, 48(5): S176–S182.

Hardwig, J. (1990). What about the family. *The Hastings Center Report*, 20(2): 5–10.

Harmsen, H., et al. (2003). When cultures meet in general practice: Intercultural differences between GPs and parents of child patients. *Patient Education and Counseling*, 51(2): 99–106.

Harpham, W. S. (2009, September 8). The value of a cancer diagnosis second opinion [Web log message]. Retrieved from: <http://www.kevinmd.com/blog/2009/09/cancer-diagnosis-second-opinion.html>.

Hart, C. N., Drotarb, D., Goric, A. and Lewin, L. (2006). Enhancing parent–provider communication in ambulatory pediatric practice. *Patient Education and Counseling*, 63: 38–46.

Hartmann, C., et al. (2007). A website to improve asthma care by suggesting patient questions for physicians: Qualitative analysis of user experiences. *Journal of Medical Internet Research*, 9: e3.

Harwood, J., and Giles, H. (2005). *Intergroup Communication: Multiple Perspectives*. New York: Peter Lang.

Harwood, J., and Roy, A. (2005). Social identity theory and mass communication research. In J. Harwood and H. Giles (eds), *Intergroup Communication: Multiple Perspectives* (pp. 189–212). New York: Peter Lang.

Harwood, J., and Sparks, L. (2003). Social identity and health: An intergroup communication approach to cancer. *Health Communication*, 15: 145–60.

Harwood, J., Giles, H., and Ryan, E. B. (1995). Aging, communication, and intergroup theory: Social identity and intergenerational communication. In J. F. Nussbaum and J. Coupland (eds), *Handbook of Communication and Aging Research* (pp. 133–59). Hillsdale, NJ: Lawrence Erlbaum.

Harwood, J., Hewstone, M., Paolini, S., and Voci, A. (2005). Grandparent–grandchild contact and attitudes towards older adults: Moderator and mediator effects. *Personality and Social Psychology Bulletin*, 31: 393–406.

Harwood, J., Soliz, J., and Lin, M.-C. (2006). Communication accommodation theory: An intergroup approach to family relationships. In D. O. Braithwaite and L. A. Baxter (eds), *Engaging Theories in Family Communication: Multiple Perspectives* (pp. 19–34). Thousand Oaks, CA: Sage.

Harzold, E., and Sparks, L. (2007). Adult child perceptions of communication and humor when the parent is diagnosed with cancer: A suggestive perspective from communication theory. *Qualitative Research Reports in Communication*, 7: 1–13.

Harzold, E., and Sparks, L. (2008). When the parent has cancer: A life span developmental approach to adult child perceptions of communication competency, humor orientation, and relational satisfaction in the older adult parent–adult child relationship. In L. Sparks, H. D. O'Hair, and G. L. Kreps, (eds), *Cancer Communication and Aging* (pp. 215–35). Cresskill, NJ: Hampton Press.

Heady, B. W., and Wearing, A. J. (1990). Subjective well-being and coping with adversity. *Social Indicators Research*, 22: 327–49.

Hecht, M. L. (1993). 2002 – a research odyssey: Toward the development of a communication theory of identity. *Communication Monographs*, 60, 76–82.

Hecht, M.L., Jackson, R. L., and Pitts, M. J. (2005). Culture: Intersections of intergroup and identity theories. In J. Harwood and H. Giles (eds), *Intergroup communication: Multiple Perspectives* (pp. 21–42). New York: Peter Lang.

Helgeson, V. S., and Cohen, S. (1999). Social support and adjustment to cancer: Reconciling descriptive, correlational, and intervention research. In R. M. Suinn and G. R. VandenBos (eds), *Cancer Patients and Their Families: Readings on Disease Course, Coping, and Psychological Interventions* (pp. 53–79). Washington DC: American Psychological Association.

Helgeson, V. S., and Gottlieb, B. H. (2000). Support groups. In S. Cohen, L. G. Underwood, and B. H. Gottlieb (eds), *Social Support Measurement and Intervention* (pp. 221–45). New York: Oxford University Press.

Helgeson, V. S., Cohen, S., Schultz, R., and Yasko, J. (2000). Group support interventions for women with breast cancer: Who benefits from what? *Health Psychology*, 19: 107–14.

Hemmerdinger, J., Stoddard, S., and Lilford, R. (2007). A systematic review of tests of empathy in medicine. *BMC Medical Education*, 24: 1–8.

Herd, D., and Grube, J. (1996). Black identity and drinking in the U. S.: A national study. *Addiction*, 91: 845–57.

Hersh, W. R., Gorman, P. N., and Sacherek, L. S. (1998). Applicability and quality of information for answering clinical questions on the web. *Journal of the American Medical Association*, 280: 1307–8.

Hesse, B. W., et al. (2005). Trust and sources of health information: The impact of the Internet and its implications for health care providers: findings from the first Health Information National Trends Survey. *Archives of Internal Medicine*, 165: 2618–24.

Hewstone, M., and Brown, R. J. (1986). Contact is not enough: An intergroup perspective on the contact hypothesis. In M. Hewstone and R. J. Brown (eds), *Contact and Conflict in Intergroup Encounters* (pp. 1–44). Oxford: Blackwell.

Hiatt, R. A., and Rimer, B. K. (1999). A new strategy for cancer control research. *Cancer Epidemiology, Biomarkers, & Prevention*, 8: 957–64.

Himes, C. L., Jordan, A. K., and Farkas, J. I. (1996). Factors influencing parental caregiving by adult women: Variations by care intensity and duration. *Research on Aging*, 18: 349–70.

Himmelstein, D., Wright, A., and Woolhandler, S. (2009). Hospital computing and the costs and quality of care: A national study. *American Journal of Medicine*, 123(1): 40–6. Available at: <http://www.ischool.drexel.edu/faculty/ssilverstein/AJM-Himmelstein-Hospital-Computing.pdf>.

Hines, S. C., Babrow, A. S., Badzek, L., and Moss, A. (2001). From coping with life to coping with death: Problematic integration for the seriously ill elderly. *Health Communication*, 13(3): 327–42.

Hofstede, G. (1991). *Culture and Organizations: Software of the Mind*. New York: McGraw Hill.

Hofstede, G. (2001). *Culture's Consequences*. Thousand Oaks, CA: Sage.

Hogan, D. P., Eggebeen, D. J., and Clogg, C. C. (1993). The structure of intergenerational exchanges in American families. *American Journal of Sociology*, 98: 1428–58.

Hogg, M., and Tindale, S. (forthcoming). Social identity, communication, and influence within small groups. In J. Harwood and H. Giles (eds), *Intergroup Communication: Multiple Perspectives*. New York: Peter Lang.

Horton, B. W., and Kline, S. L. (2007, November 15). *The Role of Communication Rituals in Models of Bereavement*. Paper presented at the annual meeting of the NCA 93rd Annual Convention, Chicago, IL. Retrieved from: <http://www.allacademic.com/meta/p_mla_apa_research_citation/1/9/3/1/7/p193176_index.html>.

Hospice Association of America. (2009). *Hospice Facts and Statistics*. Retrieved from: <http://www.nahc.org/facts/HospiceStats09.pdf>.

Hospice Foundation of America (2010). Retrieved from: <http://www.hospicefoundation.org/>.

Houston, T. K., and Allison, J. J. (2002). Users of internet health information: Differences by health status. *Journal of Medical Internet Research*, 4(2): E7.

Hovland, C. I., Janis, I. L. and Kelley, H. H. (1953) *Communications and Persuasion: Psychological Studies in Opinion Change*. New Haven, CT: Yale University Press.

Howarth, G., and Leaman, O. (eds). (2001). *Encyclopedia of Death and Dying*. London: Routledge.

Hummert, M. L., Garstka, T. A., Shaner, J. L. and Strahm, S. (1994). Stereotypes of the elderly held by the young, middle aged, and elderly adults. *Journal of Gerontology: Psychological Sciences*, 49: 240–9.

Ibrahim, S. A., Thomas, S. B., and Fine, M. J. (2003). Achieving health equity: An incremental journey. *American Journal of Public Health*, 93: 1619–21.

Ingersoll-Dayton, B., Neal, M. B., Ha, J., and Hammer, L. B. (2003). Redressing inequity in parent care among siblings. *Journal of Marriage and Family*, 65: 201–12.

Institute of Medicine (2001). *Crossing the Quality Chasm: A New Health System for the 21st Century* (Washington, D.C.: National Academies Press).

Institute of Medicine (2002a). Committee on Communication for Behavior Change in the 21st Century: Improving the Health of Diverse Populations. *Speaking of Health: Accessing Health Communication Strategies for Diverse Populations*. Washington DC: National Academy of Sciences Press.

Institute of Medicine (2002b). *Unequal Treatment: Confronting Racial and Ethnic Disparities in Health Care*. Washington DC: National Academies Press.

Institute of Medicine (2004). *Health Literacy: A Prescription to End Confusion*. Washington, DC: National Academy of Sciences Press.

Ishikawa, H., et al. (2009). Patient health literacy and patient–physician information exchange during a visit. *Family Practice*, 26: 517–23.

Jablin, F. M. (2001). Organizational entry, assimilation, and disengagement/exit. In F. M. Jablin and L. L. Putnam (eds), *The New Handbook of Organizational Communication: Advances in Theory, Research, and Methods* (pp. 732–818). Thousand Oaks, CA: Sage.

Jackson, L., and Duffy, B. (1998). *Health Communication Research: A Guide to Developments and Directions*. Westport, CT: Greenwood Press.

Jackson, L., Tudway, J. A., Giles, D., and Smith, J. (2009). An exploration of the social identity of mental health inpatient service users. *Journal of Psychiatric and Mental Health Nursing*, 16: 167–76.

Jacobs, E. A., et al. (2003). *Language Barriers in Health Care Settings: An Annotated Bibliography of the Research Literature*. Woodland Hills, CA: The California Endowment.

Janis, I. L. (1967). Effects of fear arousal on attitude change: Recent developments in theory and experimental research. In L. Berkowitz (ed.), *Advances in Experimental Social Psychology*, Vol. 3 (pp. 166–225). New York: Academic Press.

Janis, I. L., Kaye, D., and Kirschner, P. (1965). Facilitating effects of "eating-while-reading" on responsiveness to persuasive communications. *Journal of Personality and Social Psychology*, 1: 181–6.

Janz, N. K., and Becker, M. H. (1984). The health belief model: A decade later. *Health Education Quarterly*, 11: 1–47.

JCAHO (2002). *Sentinel Event Alert*, Issue 26.

Johnson, B. (2009, March 27). Free text messages save lives in Malawi. *Guardian*. Retrieved from: <http://www.guardian.co.uk/technology/2009/mar/27/mobile-phones-sms>.

Johnson, D. (1996). Helpful listening and responding. In K. M. Galvin and P. Cooper (eds), *Making Connections: Readings in Relational Communication* (pp. 91–7). Los Angeles: Roxbury.

Johnson, R. L., Roter, D., Powe, N. R., and Cooper L. A. (2004a). Patient race/ethnicity and quality of patient–physician communication during medical visits. *American Journal of Public Health*, 94: 2084–90.

Johnson, R. L., et al. (2004b). Racial and ethnic differences in patient perceptions of bias and cultural competence in health care. *Journal of General Internal Medicine*, 19: 101–10.

Joint Commission on the Accreditation of Healthcare Organizations (JCAHO). (2002). Clinical communication and patient safety. Retrieved from: <http://www.hhnmag.com/hhnmag_app/jsp/articledisplay.jsp?dcrpath=HHNMAG/PubsNewsArticle/data/2006August/0608HHN_gatefold&domain=HHNMAG>.

Jones, C. M. (1997). "That's a good sign:" Encouraging assessments as a form of social support in medically related encounters. *Health Communication*, 9: 119–53.

Jones, D. N., and Reznikoff, M. (1989). Psychosocial adjustment to a mastectomy. *Journal of Nervous and Mental Disease*, 177: 624–31.

Jones, K. C. (2008, June 18). Intel launches social networking site for family caregivers. *Information Week*. Retrieved from: <http://www.informationweek.com/news/internet/social_network/showArticle.jhtml?articleID=208700392>.

Joseph, A. E., and Hallman, B. C. (1998). Over the hill and far away: Distance as a barrier to the provision of assistance to elderly relatives. *Social Science and Medicine*, 46: 631–9.

Kahn, R. L., and Antonucci, T. C. (1980). Convoys over the life course: Attachment, roles, and social support. In P. B. Baltes and O. G. Brim (eds), *Life-span Development and Behavior* (pp. 254–83). New York: Academic Press.

Kahana, E., and Kahana, B. (2003). Patient proactivity enhancing doctor-patient-family communication in cancer prevention and care among the aged. *Patient Education and Counseling*, 50: 67–73.

Kahana, E., and Kahana, B. (2007). Healthcare partnership model of doctor–patient communication in cancer prevention and care among the aged. In D. O'Hair, G. L.

Kreps, and L. Sparks (eds), *Handbook of Communication and Cancer Care* (pp. 37–54). Cresskill, NJ: Hampton Press.

Kahneman, D., and Tversky, A. (1979). "Prospect theory:" An analysis of decision under risk. *Econometrica*, 47: 263–91.

Kahneman, D., and Tversky, A. (2000). *Choices, Values, and Frames.* Cambridge: Cambridge University Press.

Kaphingst, K. A., Rudd, R. E., DeJong, W., and Daltroy, L. H. (2005). Comprehension of information in three direct-to-consumer television prescription drug advertisements among adults with limited literacy. *Journal of Health Communication*, 10: 609–19.

Kaplan, S. H., Greenfield, S., and Ware, J. E. Jr. (1989). Assessing the effects of physician–patient interactions on the outcomes of chronic disease. *Medical Care*, 27: S110–S127.

Kaplan S. H., et al. (1995). Patient and visit characteristics related to physicians' participatory decision-making style. *Medical Care*, 33(12): 1176–87.

Karim, K., Bailey, M., and Tunna, K. (2000). Nonwhite ethnicity and the provision of specialist palliative care services: factors affecting doctors' referral patterns. *Palliative Medicine*, 14: 471–8.

Katapodi, M. C., Lee, K. A., Facione, N. C., and Dodd, M. J. (2004). Predictors of perceived breast cancer risk and the relation between perceived risk and breast cancer screening: A meta-analytic review. *Preventive Medicine*, 38: 388–403.

Katz, A. H. (1993). *Self-help in America: A Social Movement Perspective.* New York: Twayne.

Katz, A. H., and Bender, E. I. (1976). Self-help groups in Western society: History and prospects. *Journal of Applied Behavioral Science*, 12: 265–82.

Kaufman, G., and Uhlenberg, P. (1998). Effects of life course transitions on the quality of relationships between adult children and their parents. *Journal of Marriage and the Family*, 60: 924–38.

Keeley, M. P., and Yingling, J. (2007). *Final Conversations: Helping the Living and the Dying Talk to Each Other.* Acton, MA: Vanderwyk and Burnham.

Keith, D. M. (1979). Life changes and perceptions of life and death among older men and women. *Journal of Gerontology*, 34: 870–8.

Kelly, P. A., and Haidet, P. (2007). Physician overestimation of patient literacy: A potential source of health care disparities. *Patient Education and Counseling*, 66: 119–22.

Kemp, G., and Eagle, L. (2008). Shared meanings and missed opportunities? The implications of functional health literacy for social marketing interventions. *International Review on Public and Nonprofit Marketing*, 5(2): 117–28.

Kenford and Fiore (2004). Promotion tobacco cessation and relapse prevention, *Medical Clinicians North America*, 88: 1553–74.

Kessler, R. C., Mickelson, K. D., and Zhao, S. (1997). Patterns and correlates of self-help group membership in the United States. *Social Policy*, 27: 27–46.

Kidney Cancer Association (2009). *Patient Empowerment.* Retrieved from: <http://www.kidneycancer.org/knowledge/live/patient-empowerment>.

Kim, M., et al. (2000). A test of cultural model of patients' motivation for verbal communication in patient–doctor interactions. *Communication Monographs*, 67: 262–83.

Kinchen, K., et al. (2004). Referral of Patients to Specialists: Factors Affecting Choice of Specialist by Primary Care Physicians. *Annals of Family Medicine*, 2: 245–52.

Kliewer, S. (2004). Allowing spirituality into the healing process. *The Journal of Family Practice*, 53: 616–24.

Klingenberg, A., et al. (2005). Older patients' involvement in their health care: Can paper–based tools help? *Quality in Primary Care*, 13: 235–42.

Koehn, H., Desroches, N., Yum, Y., and Deagle, G. (2007). Asymmetrical talk between physicians and patients: A quantitative discourse analysis. *Canadian Journal of Communication*, 32: 417–33.

Koenig, H. G., Larson, D. B., and McCullough, M. E. (2001). *Handbook of Religion and Health*. New York: Oxford University Press.

Koerin, B. B., and Harrigan, M. P. (2002). P.S. I love you: Long-distance caregiving. *Journal of Gerontological Social Work*, 1(2): 63–81.

Kohn, L. T., Corrigan, J. M., and Donaldson, M. S. (2000). *To Err is Human: Building a Safer Health System*. Washington, DC: National Academy Press.

Kohn, P. M. (1996). On coping adaptively with daily hassles. In M. Zeidner and N. S. Endler (eds), *Handbook of Coping* (pp. 181–201). New York: John Wiley & Sons.

Korsch, B., and Harding, C. (1997). *The Intelligent Patient's Guide to the Doctor–Patient Relationship: Learning How to Talk so Your Doctor Will Listen*. New York: Oxford University Press.

Koseki, L. K. (1996). A study of utilization and satisfaction: Implications for cultural concepts and design of aging services. *Journal of Aging and Social Policy*, 8: 59–75.

Kotler, P. (1984). Social marketing of health behavior. In L. W. Frederikson, L. J. Solomon, and K. A. Brehony (eds), *Marketing Health Behavior* (pp. 23–39). New York: Plenum Press.

Kotler, P., and Roberto, E. (1989). *Social marketing*. New York: Free Press.

Koyano, W. (1996). Filial piety and intergenerational solidarity in Japan. *Australian Journal on Ageing*, 15: 51–6.

Koyano, W. (1999). Population aging, changes in living arrangement, and the new long-term care system in Japan. *Journal of Sociology and Social Welfare*, 26: 155–67.

Krause, N. (1990). Stress, support, and well-being in later life: Focusing on salient social roles. In M. A. Stephens, J. H. Crowther, S. E. Hobfoll, and D. L. Tennenbaum (eds), *Stress and Coping in Later-life Families* (pp. 71–97). New York, NY: Hemisphere Publishing Company.

Kreps, G. L. (1988). The pervasive role of information in health and health care: Implications for health communication policy. In J. Anderson (ed.), *Communication Yearbook* (pp. 238–76). Newbury Park, CA: Sage.

Kreps, G. L. (1989). Setting the agenda for health communication research and development: Scholarship that can make a difference. *Health Communication*, 1: 11–15.

Kreps, G. L. (2003a). E-health: Technology mediated health communication. *Journal of Health Psychology*, 8: 5–6.

Kreps, G. L. (2003b). Impact of communication on cancer risk, incidence, morbidity, and quality of life. *Health Communication*, 15(2): 161–9.

Kreps, G. L. (2006). Communication and racial inequities in health care. *American Behavioral Scientist*, 49: 1–15.

Kreps, G. L. (2007). A Weickian approach to public relations. In T. Hansen-Horn and B. Dostal-Neff, (eds). *Public Relations Theory* (pp. 20–30). Boston, MA: Allyn and Bacon.

Kreps, G., and O'Hair, D. (eds) (1995). *Communication and Health Outcomes*. Norwood: NJ: Hampton Press.

Kreps, G. L., and Sparks, L. (2008). Meeting the health literacy needs of vulnerable populations. *Patient Education and Counseling*, 71(3): 328–332.

Kreps, G. L., and Thornton, B. C. (1992). *Health Communication: Theory and Practice*. Prospect Heights, IL: Waveland.

Kreps, G. L., et al. (2005). Emergency/risk communication to promote public health and respond to biological threats. In M. Haider (ed.), *Global Public Health Communication: Challenges, Perspectives, and Strategies* (pp. 349–62). Sudbury, MA: Jones and Bartlett Publishers.

Kreps, G. L., Neuhauser, L., Sparks, L., and Villagran, M. (2008a). The power of community-based health communication interventions to promote cancer prevention and control for at-risk populations. *Patient Education and Counseling*, 71(3): 315–18.

Kreps, G. L., Neuhauser, L., Sparks, L., and Villagran, M. (eds) (2008b). Translational Community-Based Health Communication Interventions to Promote Cancer

Prevention and Control for Vulnerable Audiences [Special Issue]. *Patient Education and Counseling*, 71(3): 315–50.

Kreps, G. L., Villagran, M. M., and Zhao, X., (forthcoming). Development and Validation of Motivational Messages to Improve Prescription Drug Adherence. *Patient Education and Counseling*.

Kreuter, M. W., and Haughton, L. T. (2006). Integrating culture into health information for African American women. *American Behavioral Scientist*, 49: 794–811.

Kreuter, M. W., and Strecher, V. J. (1995). Changing inaccurate perceptions of health risk: Results from a randomized trial. *Health Psychology*, 14: 56–63.

Kreuter, M., Farrell, D., Olevitch, L., and Brennan, L. (2000). *Tailoring health messages: Customizing Communication with Computer Technology*. Mahwah, NJ: Lawrence Erlbaum.

Krieger, N. (1990). Racial and gender discrimination: Risk factors for high blood pressure? *Social Science and Medicine*, 30: 1273–81.

Kripalani, Sunil, Paasche-Orlow, M. K., Parker, R. M., and Saha, S. (2006). Advancing the field of health literacy. *Journal of General Internal Medicine*, 21: 804–6.

Kruijver, I. P., Kerkstra, A., Bensing, J. M., and Van de Wiel, H. B. (2001). Communication skills of nurses during interactions with simulated cancer patients. *Journal of Advanced Nursing*, 34(6): 772–9.

Ku, L., and Flores, G. (2005). Pay now or pay later: providing interpreter services in health care. *Health Affairs*, 24: 435–44.

Kubler-Ross, E. (1969). *On Death and Dying: What the Dying Have to Teach Doctors, Nurses, Clergy, and Their Own Families*. New York: Routledge.

Kulis, S. (1987). Socially mobile daughters and sons of the elderly: Mobility effects within the family revisited. *Journal of Marriage and the Family*, 49: 421–33.

Kundrat, A. L., and Nussbaum, J. F. (2003). The impact of invisible illness on identity and contextual age across the life span. *Health Communication*, 15: 331–47.

Kutner, M., Greenberg, E., Jin, Y., and Paulsen, C. (2006). *The Health Literacy of America's Adults: Results from the 2003 National Assessment of Adult Literacy*. (US Department of Education and National Center for Education Statistics Publication No. 2006–483).

Kuzsler, P. (2000). A question of duty: Common law legal issues resulting from physician response to unsolicited patient email inquiries. *Journal of Medical Internet Research*, 2: e17.

La Gaipa, J. J. (1990). The negative effects of informal support systems. In S. Duck and R. C. Silver (eds), *Personal Relationships and Social Support* (pp. 122–39). Newbury Park, CA: Sage.

Laizner, A. M., Yost, L. M., Barg, F. K., and McCorkle, R. (1993). Needs of family caregivers of persons with cancer: A review. *Seminars in Oncology Nursing*, 9: 114–120.

Lantz, P. M., et al. (1995). Breast and cervical cancer screening in a low-income managed care sample: The efficacy of physician letters and phone calls. *American Journal of Public Health*, 85: 834–6.

LaRocca, J., House, J., and French, J. R. (1980). Social support, occupational health, and stress. *Journal of Health and Social Behavior*, 21: 201–18.

Larsen, A. (2009, October 14). Health care reform's effect on medical negligence cases [Web log message]. Retrieved from: <http://ezinearticles.com/?Health-Care-Reforms-Effect-on-Medical-Negligence-Cases&id=3093436>.

Lasswell, H. D. (1948). The structure and function of communication in society. In L. Bryson (ed.), *The Communication of Ideas* (pp. 32–5). New York: Institute for Religious and Social Studies.

Lawton, J. (2000). *The Dying Process: Patients' Experiences of Palliative Care*. London: Routledge.

Lederer, R. (2000). *The Bride of Anguished English: A Bonanza of Bloopers, Blunders, Botchers, and Boo Boos*. New York: St Martin's Press.

Lee, G. R., Netzer, J. K., and Coward, R. T. (1995). Family structure and filial responsibility expectations among older parents. *Journal of Clinical Geropsychology*, 1: 133–45.

Leets, L. (2001). Response to Internet hate sites: Is speech too free in cyberspace? *Communication Law and Policy*, 6: 287–317.

Lefebvre, R. C., and Flora, J. A. (1988). Social marketing and public health intervention. *Health Education Quarterly*, 15: 299–315.

Lehman, D. R., Ellard, J. H., and Wortman, C. B. (1986). Social support for the bereaved: Recipients' and providers' perspectives on what is helpful. *Journal of Consulting and Clinical Psychology*, 54: 438–46.

Leman, H. (2009, November 5). Maneuvering medical institutions through the wild waters of social media: A talk with John Sharp of the Cleveland Clinic [Web log message]. Retrieved from: <http://significantscience.com/2009/11/05/maneuvering-medical-institutions-through-the-wild-waters-of-social-media-a-talk-with-john-sharp-of-the-cleveland-clinic/>.

Lennon, A., Gallois, C., Owen, N., and McDermott, L. (2005). Young women as smokers and nonsmokers: A qualitative social identity approach. *Qualitative Health Research*, 15: 1345–59.

Lepore, S. J., Allen, K. A. M., and Evans, G. W. (1993). Social support lowers cardiovascular reactivity to an acute stressor. *Psychosomatic Medicine*, 55: 518–24.

Lester, D. (1992). The stigma against dying and suicidal patients: A replication of Richard Kalish's study twenty-five years later. *Omega: Journal of Death and Dying*, 26: 71–5.

Lett, J. E., and Scherger, J. E. (2007). *Health IT Done Right Improves Care* [e-letter]. Retrieved from: <http://www.annfammed.org/cgi/eletters/5/4/320#5991>.

Levine, B.A., et al. (2009). Communication plays a critical role in web based monitoring. *Journal of Diabetes Science and Technology*, 3(3): 461–7.

Leventhal, H. (1970). Findings and theory in the study of fear communications. In L. Berkowitz (ed.), *Advances in Experimental Social Psychology* (Vol. 5, pp. 119–86). New York: Academic Press.

Leviss, J. (2009, December 29). Add "meaningful use" for patients [Web log message]. Retrieved from: <http://www.modernhealthcare.com/article/20091229/REG/312289886#>.

Levy, B. (1996). Improving memory in old age through implicit self-stereotyping. *Journal of Personality and Social Psychology*, 71: 1092–1107.

Levy, B. R., Zonderman, A. B., Slade, M. D., and Ferrucci, L. (2009). Age stereotypes held earlier in life predict cardiovascular events in later life. *Psychological Science*, 20(3): 296–8.

Lewis, D. (2009, March 9). It's the right call for some. *Los Angeles Times*, pp. E1, E3.

Lin, G., and Rogerson, P. (1995). Elderly parents and the geographic availability of their adult children. *Research on Aging*, 17: 303–31.

Linden, M., and Godemann, F. (2007). The difference between lack of insight and dysfunctional health beliefs in schizophrenia. *Psychopathology*, 40: 236–41.

Lindquist, A., et al. (2008). The use of the personal digital assistant (PDA) among personnel and students in health care: A review. *Journal of Medical Internet Research*, 10: e31.

Litwak, E. (1985). *Helping the Elderly: The Complementary Rules of Informal Networks and Formal Systems*. New York: Guilford Press.

Litwak, E., and Meyer, H. (1966). A balanced theory of coordination between bureaucratic organizations and community primary groups. *Administrative Science Quarterly*, 11: 31–58.

Litwak, E., and Kulis, S. (1987). Technology, proximity, and measures of kin support. *Journal of Marriage and the Family*, 49: 649–61.

Louis, M. R. (1980). Surprise and sensemaking: What newcomers experience in entering unfamiliar organizational settings. *Administrative Science Quarterly*, 25: 226–51.

Luszczynska, A., and Schwarzer, R. (2003). Planning and self–efficacy in the adoption and maintenance of breast self-examination: A longitudinal study on self-regulatory cognitions. *Psychology and Health*, 18: 93–108.

Lynn, J. (2000). Preface. In K. L. Braun, J. H. Pietsch, and P. L. Blanchette (eds), *Cultural Issues in End-of-Life Decision Making* (pp. ix–xi). Thousand Oaks, CA: Sage.

Lynn, J. (2001). Serving patients who may die soon and their families: The role of hospice and other services. *Journal of the American Medical Association*, 285(7): 925–32.

Lynn, J. and Goldstein, N. (2003). Advance care planning for fatal chronic illness: Avoiding commonplace errors and unwarranted suffering. *Annals of Internal Medicine*, 138(10): 812–18.

Maass, A., Salvi, D., Arcuri, L., and Semin, G. (1989). Language use in intergroup contexts: The linguistic intergroup bias. *Journal of Personality and Social Psychology*, 57: 981–93.

McCubbin, M. A., and McCubbin, H. I. (1991) Family stress theory and assessment: The resiliency model of family stress, adjustment, and adaptation. In H. I. McCubbin and A. I. Thompson (eds), *Family Assessment Inventories for Research and Practice* (pp. 3–32). Madison, WI: University of Wisconsin.

MacDonald, L. D., and Anderson, H. R. (1984). Stigma in patients with rectal cancer: A community study. *Journal of Epidemiology and Community Health*, 38: 284–90.

McGee, M. K. (2009, November 13). Health care IT gets personal. *Information Week*. Retrieved from: <http://www.informationweek.com/news/healthcare/EMR/showArticle.jhtml?articleID=221601548>.

McGee, R. (1999). Does stress cause cancer? There's no good evidence of a relation between stressful events and cancer. *British Medical Journal*, 319(7216): 1015–16.

McGorry, S. Y. (1999). An investigation of expectations and perceptions of health–care services with a Latino population. *Journal of Health Care Quality Assurance*, 12: 190–7.

Mackie, D. M. and Smith, E. R. (2002). *From Prejudice to Intergroup Emotions: Differentiated Reactions to Social Groups*. New York: Psychology Press.

McLuhan, M. (1964). *Understanding Media: The Extensions of Man*. New York: Signet.

MacMillan, S. C., and Small, B. J. (2002). Symptom distress and quality of life in patients with cancer newly admitted to hospice home care. *Oncology Nursing Forum*, 29: 1421–8.

McNeill, P. M., and Walton, M. (2002). Medical harm and the consequences of error for doctors. *Medical Journal of Australia*, 176(5): 222–5.

McWilliam, C. L. (2009). Patients, persons or partners? Involving those with chronic disease in their care. *Chronic Illness*. Retrieved from: <http://chi.sagepub.com/cgi/content/abstract/1742395309349315v1>.

McWilliam, C. L., Brown, J. B., and Stewart, M. (2000). Breast cancer patients' experiences of patient–doctor communication: A working relationship. *Patient Education and Counseling*, 39(2–3):191–204.

Maddox, P. (2002). Ethics and the brave new world of e-health. *The Online Journal of Issues in Nursing*, 6(3). Retrieved from: <http://www.doaj.org/doaj?func=abstract&id=116810>.

Magen, R., and Glajchen, M. (1999). Cancer support groups: Client outcome and the context of group process. *Research on Social Work Practice*, 9(5): 362–75.

Maguire P. (1998). Breaking bad news. *European Journal of Surgical Oncology*, 24: 188–99.

Maheswaran, D., and Chaiken, S. (1991). Promoting systematic processing in low–motivation settings: Effect of incongruent information on processing and judgment. *Journal of Personality and Social Psychology*, 61: 13–25.

Maheu, M. M., Whitten, P., and Allen, A. (2001). *E-health, Telehealth, and Telemedicine: A Guide to Start-up and Success*. New York: Jossey-Bass.

Maibach, E. W., and Cotton, D. (1995). Moving people to behavior change: A staged social cognitive approach to message design. In E. W. Maibach and R. L. Parrott (eds), *Designing Health Messages: Approaches from Communication Theory and Public Health Practice* (pp. 41–64). Newbury Park, CA: Sage.

Maibach, E. W., Kreps, G. L., and Bonaguro, E. W. (1996). Developing strategic communication campaigns for HIV/AIDS prevention. In S. Ratzan (ed.), *AIDS: Effective Communication for the 90s* (pp. 15–35). Washington, DC: Taylor and Francis.

Manderson, L. (1999). Gender, normality and the post-surgical body. *Anthropology and Medicine*, 6: 381–94.

Mandl, K. D., Szolovits, P. and Kohane, I. S. (2001). Public standards and patients' control: How to keep electronic medical records accessible but private. *British Medical Journal*, 322(7281): 283–7.

Marchand, L., and Kushner, K. (2004). Death pronouncements: Using the teachable moment in end-of-life care residency training. *Journal of Palliative Medicine*, 7: 80–4.

Marshall, A. A. (1993). Whose agenda is it anyway?: Training medical residents in patient–centered interviewing techniques. In E. B. Ray (ed.), *Case Studies in Health Communication* (pp. 15–30). Hillsdale, NJ: Lawrence Erlbaum Associates.

Martin, D. K., Emanuel, L. L., and Singer, P. A. (2000). Planning for the end of life. *Lancet*, 356: 1672–6.

Martinez, J. M. (1996). The interdisciplinary team. In D. C. Sheehan and W. B. Forman (eds), *Hospice and Palliative Care: Concepts and Practices* (pp. 21–9). Sudbury, MA: Jones and Bartlett Publishers.

Mastro, D. (2003). A social identity approach to understanding the impact of television messages. *Communication Monographs*, 70: 98–113.

Mathieson, C. M., et al. (1996). Caring for head and neck oncology patients: Does social support lead to better quality of life? *Canadian Family Physician*, 42: 1712–20.

Maynard, D. W. (1991). Bearing bad news in clinical settings. In B. Dervin and M. J. Voigt (eds), *Progress in Communication Sciences*, (Vol. 10, pp. 143–72). Norwood, NJ: Ablex.

Mears, J. B. (1997). The cultural construction of breast cancer. *Dissertation Abstracts International Section A: Humanities and Social Sciences*, 58(6-A): 2273.

Medline Plus (2010). *Hospice Care*. Retrieved from: <http://www.nlm.nih.gov/medlineplus/hospicecare.html>.

Mehrabian, A. (1981). *Silent Messages: Implicit Communication of Emotions and Attitudes*. Belmont, CA: Wadsworth.

Mercer, S. O. (1994). Navajo elders in a reservation nursing home: Health status profile. *Journal of Geronotological Social Work*, 23: 3–29.

Messigner-Rapport, B. J., Baum, E. E., and Smith, M. L. (2009). Advance care planning: Beyond the living will. *Cleveland Clinic Journal of Medicine*, 76: 276–85.

Meyer, G., and Dearing, J. W. (1996). Respecifying the social marketing model for unique populations. *Social Marketing Quarterly* 3 (Winter): 44–52.

Meyerowitz, B. E., and Chaiken, S. (1987). The effect of message framing on breast self-examination attitudes, intentions, and behaviors. *Journal of Personality and Social Psychology*, 52(3): 500–11.

Meyers, J. L., and Gray, L. N. (2001). The relationships between family primary caregiver characteristics and satisfaction with hospice care, quality of life, and burden. *Oncology Nursing Forum*, 28: 73–82.

Michie, S., and Abraham, C. (2004). Interventions to change health behaviours: Evidence-based or evidence-inspired? *Psychology and Health*, 19: 29–49.

Michigan Department of Community Health (2000). Three-month-old baby dies of acute hepatitis B. *Michigan Immunization Update*, 7(2): 1–2.

Mickus, M. A., and Luz, C. C. (2002). Televisits: Sustaining long distance family relationships among institutionalized elders through technology. *Aging & Mental Health*, 6: 387–96.

Miller, L. C., Berg, J. H., and Archer, R. L. (1983). Openers: Individuals who elicit intimate self-disclosure. *Journal of Personality and Social Psychology*, 44: 1234–44.

Miller, V. D., and Jablin, F. M. (1991). Information seeking during organizational entry: Influences, tactics, and a model of the process. *Academy of Management Review*, 16: 92–120.

Mishel, M. (1988). Uncertainty in illness. *Image: The Journal of Nursing of Scholarship*, 20: 225–32.

Mishel, M., and Braden, C. J. (1988). Antecedents of uncertainty in illness. *Nursing Research*, 27: 98–127.

Mishel, M., and Clayton, M. F. (2003). Uncertainty in illness theories. In M. J. Smith, P. Liehr (eds) *Middle Range Theory in Advanced Practiced Nursing* (pp. 25–48). New York: Springer.

Mishler, E. G. (1984). The discourse of medicine. *Culture, Medicine and Psychiatry*, 12: 249–56.

Mishra, D. K., Alreja, S., Sengar, K.S., and Singh, A. R. (2009). Insight and its relationship with stigma. *India Psychiatry Journal*, 18: 39–42.

Mitchell, M. M. (2000). Motivated, but not able? The effects of positive and negative mood on persuasive message processing. *Communication Monographs*, 67: 215–25.

Mitchell, M. M., Brown, K. M., Morris Villagran, M. and Villagran, P. D. (2001). The effects of anger, sadness and happiness on persuasive message processing: A test of the negative state relief model. *Communication Monographs*, 68: 347–59.

Mok, B. H. (2001). Cancer self-help groups in China: A study of individual change, perceived benefit, and community impact. *Small Group Research*, 32: 115–32.

Mok, E., and Martinson, I. (2000). Empowerment of Chinese patients with cancer through self-help groups in Hong Kong. *Cancer Nursing*, 23: 206–13.

Mold, J. W. (1995). An alternative conceptualization of health and health care: Its implications for geriatrics and gerontology. *Educational Gerontology*, 21: 85–101.

Moody, H. R. (1994). *Aging: Concepts and Controversies.* Thousand Oaks, CA: Pine Forge.

Moore, D. L., Hausknecht, D., and Thamodaran, K. (1986). Time compression, response opportunity, and persuasion. *The Journal of Consumer Research*, 13: 85–99.

Morgan, S. E. and Miller, J. K. (2002). Beyond the organ donor card: The effect of knowledge, attitudes, and values on willingness to communicate about organ donation to family members. *Health Communication*, 14: 121–34.

Morman, M. T. (2000). The influence of fear appeals, message design, and masculinity on men's motivation to perform the testicular self-exam. *Journal of Applied Communication Research*, 28(2): 91–116.

Morrow, A. (2009, August 19). How will health care reform affect end-of-life care? [Web log message]. Retrieved from: <http://dying.about.com/od/ethicsandchoices/f/health_reform_EOL.ht>.

Moyad, M. A. (2003). Bladder cancer prevention. Part I: What do I tell my patients about lifestyle changes and dietary supplements? *Current Opinion in Urology*, 13: 363–78.

Mossakowski, K. N. (2003). Coping with perceived discrimination: Does ethnic identity protect mental health? *Journal of Health and Social Behavior*, 44: 318–31.

Mouton, C. P. (2000). Cultural and religious issues for African Americans. In K. L. Braun, J. H. Pietsch, and P. L. Blanchette (eds), *Cultural Issues in End-of-Life Decision Making* (pp. 71–82). Thousand Oaks, CA: Sage.

Mullens, A. B., McCaul, K. D., Erickson, S. C., and Sandgren, A. K. (2004). Coping after cancer: Risk perceptions, worry, and health behaviors among colorectal cancer survivors. *Psycho-Oncology*, 13: 367–76.

Nail, L. M. (2002). Fatigue in patients with cancer. *Oncology Nursing Forum*, 29: 537–46.

Napoli, P. M. (2001). Consumer use of medical information from electronic and paper media. In R. E. Rice, and J. E. Katz (eds), *The Internet and Health Communication: Experiences and Expectations* (pp. 79–98). Thousand Oaks, CA: Sage Publications.

National Alliance for Caregiving and the Metlife Mature Market Institute (2004). *Miles Away: The Metlife Study of Long-distance Caregiving*. Bethesda, MD: NAC and New York: MMMI.

National Cancer Institute. (1998, June). *How the Public Perceives, Processes, and Interprets Risk Information: Findings from Focus Group Research* (Report No.: POS-T086). Bethesda, MD: Office of Cancer Communications.

National Cancer Institute (2005). *The Health Information National Trends Survey (HINTS)*. Retrieved from: <http://hints.cancer.gov/docs/HINTS-Briefing-12-18-03.pdf>.

National Center for Education Statistics (2003). *National Assessment of Adult Literacy*. Retrieved from: <http://nces.ed.gov/naal/index.asp>.

National Center for Health Statistics (1994). *Health, United States 1993*. Hyattsville, MD: United States Department of Health and Human Services.

National Center for Health Statistics (2000). *Health, United States, 2000*. Hyattsville, MD: United States Department of Health and Human Services.

National Center on Minority Health and Health Disparities. (2009). *National Institute of Health*. Retrieved from: <http://ncmhd.nih.gov/>.

National Family Caregivers Association (2005). *Who are Family Caregivers?* Retrieved August 27, 2005, from: <http://www.thefamilycaregiver.org/who/>.

National Hospice and Palliative Care Organization (2009). Advancing care at the end of life. Retrieved from: <http://www.nhpco.org/>.

National Network of Libraries of Medicine (2010). *Health Literacy*. Retrieved from: <http://nnlm.gov/outreach/consumer/hlthlit.html>.

Nelson, A. (2002). Unequal treatment: confronting racial and ethnic disparities in health care. *Journal of the National Medical Association*, 94: 666–8.

Neuhauser, L., and Kreps, G. L. (2003). Rethinking communication in the e-health era. *Journal of Health Psychology*, 8: 7–23.

New Hampshire Health Information Center. (2009). *NH Health Cost*. Retrieved from: <http://www.nhhealthcost.org/default.aspx>.

Ng, S. H., Giles, H., and Moody, J. (1991). Information-seeking triggered by age. *International Journal of Aging and Human Development*, 33: 269–77.

Nicoll, L. H. (2002). When there's little time left. *Journal of Hospice and Palliative Nursing*, 4: 4–5.

Nielsen-Bohlman, L. (2004). *Understanding Health Literacy: Implications for Medicine and Public Health*. Chicago, IL: American Medical Association.

Nielsen-Bohlman, L., Panzer, A. M., and Kindig, D. A. (2004). *Health Literacy: A Prescription to End Confusion*. Washington, DC: National Academies Press.

Noone, I., Crowe, M., Pillay, I., and O'Keeffe, S. T. (2000). Telling the truth about cancer: Views of elderly patients and their relatives. *Irish Medical Journal*, 93(4): 104–5.

Nordin, A., et al. (2001). Do elderly cancer patients care about cure? *Gynecological Oncology*, 81(3): 447–55.

Norman, N. M., and Tedeschi, J. T. (1989). Self-presentation, reasoned action, and adolescents' decisions to smoke cigarettes. *Journal of Applied Social Psychology*, 19: 543–58.

Northouse, P. G., and Northouse, L. L. (1988). Communication and cancer: Issues confronting patients, health professionals, and family members. *Journal of Psychosocial Oncology*, 5(3): 17–46.

Northouse, L. L., and Northouse, P. G. (1998). *Health Communication: Strategies for Health Professionals*, 3rd edn. Stamford, CT: Appleton & Lange.

Nussbaum, J. F. (1989). Directions for research within health communication. *Health Communication*, 1: 35–40.

Nussbaum, J. F., and Fisher, C. F. (2009). A communication model for the competent delivery of geriatric medicine. *Journal of Language and Social Psychology*, 28: 190–208.

Nussbaum, J. F., Baringer, D., and Kundrat, A. (2003). Health, communication, and aging: Cancer and older adults. *Health Communication*, 15: 185–92.

Nussbaum, J. F., Bergstrom, M., and Sparks, L. (1996). The institutionalized elderly: Interactive implications of long-term care. In E. Ray (ed.), *Communication and Disenfranchisement: Social Health Issues and Implications* (pp. 219–32). Mahwah, NJ: Lawrence Erlbaum Associates.

Nussbaum, J. F., Pecchioni, L., Baringer, D., and Kundrat, A. L. (2002). Lifespan communication. In W. B. Gudykunst (ed.), *Communication Yearbook 26* (pp. 366–89). Mahwah, NJ: Erlbaum.

Nussbaum, J. F., Pecchioni, L., Robinson, J. D., and Thompson, T. (2000). *Communication and Aging* (2nd edn). Mahwah, NJ: Lawrence Erlbaum Associates, Inc.

Nussbaum, J. F., Sparks, L., and Bergstrom, M. (1996). Elder care: Different paths within an extended American family. In E. Ray (ed.), *Case Studies in Communication and Disenfranchisement: Applications to Social Health Issues* (pp. 99–108). Mahwah, NJ: Lawrence Erlbaum Associates.

O'Connor, A. (2004, April 27). Take two aspirin, e-mail me tomorrow. *The New York Times*. Retrieved from: <http://www.nytimes.com/2004/04/27/health/take-two-aspirin-e-mail-me-tomorrow.html?pagewanted=1>.

O'Donoghue, F. (2009). *Focus on Death and Dying. Studies*. Retrieved from: <http://www.studiesirishreview.ie/j/page72>.

O'Hair, H. D., and Sparks, L. (2008). Relational agency in life threatening illnesses. In K. Wright and S. D. Moore (eds), *Applied Health Communication* (pp. 271–89). Cresskill, NJ: Hampton Press.

O'Hair, H. D., Kreps, G. L., and Sparks, L. (2007). Conceptualizing cancer care and communication. In H. D. O'Hair, L. Sparks, and G. L. Kreps (eds), *Handbook of Communication and Cancer Care* (pp. 1–12). Cresskill, NJ: Hampton Press.

O'Hair, D., Scannell, D., and Thompson, S. (Forthcoming.). Agency through narrative: Patients managing cancer care in a challenging environment. In L. Harter, P. Japp, and C. Beck (eds), *Constructing Our Health: The Implications of Narrative for Enacting Illness and Wellness*. Mahwah, NJ: Erlbaum.

O'Hair, H. D., Sparks, L., and Kreps, G. L., (eds). (2007). *Handbook of Communication and Cancer Care*. Cresskill, NJ: Hampton Press.

O'Hair, H. D., Thompson, S., and Sparks, L. (2005). Negotiating cancer care through agency. In E. B. Ray (ed.). *Health Communication in Practice: A Case Study Approach* (pp. 81–94). Mahwah, NJ: Erlbaum.

O'Hair, H. D., et al. (2003). Cancer survivorship and agency model: Implications for patient choice, decision making, and influence. *Health Communication*, 15: 193–202.

Oakes, P. J., Haslam, S. A., and Turner, J. C. (1994). *Stereotyping and Social Reality*. Oxford: Blackwell.

Office of Disease Prevention and Health Promotion (2006). Health people 2010 midcourse review. Retrieved from: <http://www.healthypeople.gov/Data/midcourse/pdf/fa11.pdf>.

Office of Minority Health (2005).National study of culturally and linguistically appropriate services in managed care organizations. Retrieved from: <http://www.omhrc.gov/cultural/MCOCLAS-1 Final Report Main1.pdf>.

Ofri, D. (2009, October 20). Medicine in translation [Web log message]. Retrieved from: <http://www.psychologytoday.com/blog/medicine-in-translation/200910/medicine-in-translation>.

Ogden, J., and Nicoll, M. (1997). Risk and protective factors: An integration of the epidemiological and psychological approaches to adolescent smoking. *Addiction Research*, 5(5): 367–77.

Ojanlatva, A., et al. (1997). The use of problem-based learning in dealing with cultural minority groups. *Patient Education and Counseling*, 31: 171–6.

Oldenburg, B., and Parcel, G. S. (2002). Diffusion of innovations. In K. Glanz, B. K. Rimer, and F. M. Lewis (eds), *Health Behavior and Health Education: Theory, Research, and Practice* (3rd edn, pp. 312–34). San Francisco: Josey-Bass.

Ong, L., et al. (1998). The Roter Interaction Analysis System (RIAS) in oncological consultations: Psychometric properties. *Psycho-oncology*, 7: 387–401.

Ong, L., Visser, M., Lammes, F., and de Haes, J. (2000). Doctor–patient communication and cancer patients' quality of life and satisfaction. *Patient Education and Counseling*, 41: 145–56.

OPTN. (2005). The organ procurement and transplantation network: Waiting list removal reasons by year. Retrieved April 30, 2005. Available from: <http://www.optn.org/latest-Data/rptData.asp>.

Orbe, M. P. (1998). From the standpoint(s) of traditionally muted groups: Explicating a co-cultural communication theoretical model. *Communication Theory*, 8: 1–26.

Organizing for America. (2010). The Obama Plan. Retrieved from: <http://www.barackobama.com/issues/healthcare/>.

Paasche-Orlow, M. K. (2005). The Challenges of Informed Consent for Low-Literate Populations. In J. G. Schwartzberg, J. B. Van Geest, and C. C. Wang (eds), *Understanding Health Literacy* (pp. 119–40). Chicago, IL: AMA Press.

Paasche-Orlow, M. K., et al. (2005a). The prevalence of limited health literacy. *Journal of General Internal Medicine*, 20: 175–84.

Paasche-Orlow, et al. (2005b). Tailored education may reduce health literacy disparities in asthma self-management. *American Journal of Respiratory and Critical Care Medicine*, 172: 980–6.

Paasche-Orlow, M. K., Schillinger, D., Greene, S. M., and Wagner, E. H. (2006). How health care systems can begin to address the challenge of limited literacy. *Journal of General Internal Medicine*, 21: 884–8.

Paloutzian, R. F., and Kirkpatrick, L. K. (1995). Introduction: The scope of religious influences on personal and societal well-being. *Journal of Social Issues*, 51(2): 1–11.

Panke, J. T. (2002). Difficulties in managing pain at the end of life. *American Journal of Nursing*, 102: 26–33.

Pargament, K. I. (1990). *The Psychology of Religion and Coping: Theory, Research, and Practice*. New York: Guilford Press.

Park, C. L., Zlateva, I., and Blank, T. O. (2009). Self-identity after cancer: "survivor," "victim," "patient," and "person with cancer." *Journal of General Internal Medicine*, 24: 430–5.

Parker, R., and Aggleton, P. (2003). HIV and AIDS-related stigma and discrimination: A conceptual framework and implications for action. *Social Science and Medicine*, 57: 13–24.

Parker, R. M., and Davis, T. C. (2006). *To Err really is Human: Misunderstanding Medication Labels*. Federal Drug Administration. Retrieved from: <http://www.fda.gov/ohrms/dockets/ac/06/slides/2006-4230s1_01_02_Davis%20and%20Parker.ppt>.

Parrott, R. (ed.). (2004). Religious faith, spirituality, and health communication [Special Issue]. *Health Communication*, 16(1): 1–130.

Parsons, T. (1951). *The Social System*. Glencoe, IL: The Free Press.

Partnership for Clear Health Communication (2006). Clear health communication in action. *Journal of General Internal Medicine*, 21: 847–51.

Patt, M. R., et al. (2003). Doctors who are using e-mail with their patients: A qualitative exploration. *Journal of Medical Internet Research*, 5: e9.

Patterson, R., Neuhouser, M., and Hedderson, M. (2003). Cancer survivor's lifestyle changes. *Nutrition Research Newsletter*, 22: 5–6.

Pecchioni, L. L., and Nussbaum, J. F. (2000). The influence of autonomy and paternalism on communicative behaviors in mother–daughter relationships prior to dependency. *Health Communication*, 12: 317–38.

Pecchioni, L. L., and Nussbaum, J. F. (2001). Mother–daughter adult discussions of caregiving prior to dependency: Exploring conflicts among European-American women. *The Journal of Family Communication*, 1: 133–50.

Pecchioni, L., and Sparks, L. (2007). Health information sources of individuals with cancer and their family members. *Health Communication*, 21: 143–51.

Pecchioni, L., Ota, H., and Sparks, L. (2004). Cultural issues in communication and aging (2nd edn). In J. F. Nussbaum and J. Coupland (eds), *Handbook of Communication and Aging Research* (pp. 167–207). Mahwah, NJ: Erlbaum.

Pecchioni, L., Wright, K., and Nussbaum, J. F. (2005). *Life-span Communication*. Mahwah, NJ: Lawrence Erlbaum.

Pecchioni, L., et al. (2008). Investigating cancer and ageing from a cultural perspective. In L. Sparks, H. D. O'Hair, and G. L. Kreps, (eds), *Cancer Communication and Aging* (pp.239–57). Cresskill, NJ: Hampton Press.

Pechmann, C. (2001). A comparison of health communication models: Risk learning versus stereotype priming. *Media Psychology*, 3(2): 189–210.

Pederson, L. L., Koval, J. J., and O'Connor, K. (1997). Are psychosocial factors related to smoking in grade-6 students? *Addictive Behaviors*, 22: 169–81.

Perloff, R. M., et al. (2006). Doctor–patient communication, cultural competence, and minority health. *American Behavioral Scientist*, 49: 835–52.

Peters, L., den Boer, D. J., Kok, G., and Schaalma, H. P. (1994). Public reactions towards people with AIDS: An attributional analysis. *Patient Education and Counseling*, 24: 323–35.

Peters, E., Lipkus, I., and Defenbach, M. (2006). The functions of affect in health communications and in the construction of health preferences. *Journal of Communication*, 56, 140–52.

Petronio, S. (2002). *Boundaries of Privacy: Dialectics of Disclosure*. Albany, NY: SUNY Press.

Petronio, S. (2006). Impact of medical mistakes: Navigating work–family boundaries for physicians and their families. *Communication Monographs*, 73: 463–7.

Pettigrew, T. (1998). Intergroup contact theory. *Annual Review of Psychology*, 49: 65–85.

Petty, R. E., Barden, J., and Wheeler, C. M. (2002). The elaboration likelihood model of persuasion: Health promotions that yield sustained behavioral change. In R. J. DiClemente, R. A. Crosby, and M. C. Kegler (eds), *Emerging Theories in Health Promotion Practice and Research: Strategies for Improving Public Health* (pp. 71–99). San Francisco: Josey-Bass.

Petty, R. E., and Cacioppo, J. T. (1986). The elaboration likelihood model of persuasion. *Advances in Hydroscience*, 19: 124–205.

Petty, R. E., Cacioppo, J. T., and Goldman, R. (1981). Personal involvement as a determinant of argument-based persuasion. *Journal of Personality and Social Psychology*, 41: 847–55.

Petty, R. E., and Wegener, D. T. (1999). The elaboration likelihood model: Current status and controversies. In S. Chaiken, and Y. Trope (eds), *Dual-process Theories in Social Psychology* (pp. 37–72). New York: Guilford Press.

Petty, R. E., Wells, G. L., and Brock, T. C. (1976). Distraction can enhance or reduce yielding to propaganda: Thought disruption versus effort justification. *Journal of Personality and Social Psychology*, 34: 874–84.

Pew Research (2009, June 11). The shared search for health information on the internet. *Pew Internet and American Life Project*. Retrieved from: <http://pewresearch.org/pubs/1248/americans-look-online-for-health-information>.

Phillips, D. R. (2000). *Ageing in the Asia-Pacific Region: Issues, Policies and Future Trends*. London: Routledge.

Phinney, J. S. (1990). Ethnic identity in adolescents and adults: Review of research. *Psychological Bulletin*, 108: 499–514.

Pho, K. (2009, December 15). *How Twitter Will Impact Health Care in 2010* [Web log message]. Retrieved from: <http://www.kevinmd.com/blog/2009/12/twitter-impact-health-care-2010.html>.

Pierce, G. R., Sarason, I. G., and Sarason, B. R. (1996). Coping and social support. In M. Zeidner and N. S. Endler (eds), *Handbook of Coping* (pp. 434–51). New York: John Wiley & Sons, Inc.

Pitts, M. J., et al. (2009). Dialectical tensions underpinning family farm succession planning. *Journal of Applied Communication Research*, 37: 59–79.

Pitula, C. R., and Daugherty, S. R. (1995). Sources of social support and conflict in hospitalized depressed women. *Nursing and Health*, 18: 325–32.

Pollard, B. (2009, December 7). *Why Doctors Need To Take Reputation Management Seriously* [Web log message]. Retrieved from: <http://ow.ly/JUNP>.

Pomerantz, A. M., Fehr, B. J., and Ende, J. (1997). When supervising physicians see patients: Strategies used in difficult situations. *Human Communication Research*, 23(4), 589–615.

Postmes, T., and Baym, N. (forthcoming). Intergroup dimensions of the internet. In J. Harwood and H. Giles (eds), *Intergroup Communication: Multiple Perspectives*. New York: Peter Lang.

Postmes, T., and Spears, R. (1998). Deindividuation and antinormative behavior: A meta-analysis. *Psychological Bulletin*, 123: 238–59.

Postmes, T., Spears, R., and Lea, M. (1998). Breaching or building social boundaries? SIDE-effects of computer-mediated communication. *Communication Research*, 25: 689–715.

Poulson, J. (1998). Impact of cultural differences in care of the terminally ill. In N. MacDonald (ed.), *Palliative Medicine: A Case-based Manual* (pp. 244–52). New York: Oxford University Press.

Powell, C. K., and Kripalani, S. (2005). Brief report: Resident recognition of low literacy a risk factor in hospital remission. *Journal of General Internal Medicine*, 20: 1042–4.

Prochaska, J. O., DiClemente, C. C., and Norcross, J. C. (1992). In search of how people change. *American Psychologist*, 47: 1102–14.

Query, J. L., and Kreps, G. L. (1996). Testing a relational model for health communication competence among caregivers for individuals with Alzheimer's disease. *Journal of Health Psychology*, 1: 335–51.

Query, J. L., and Wright, K. B. (2003). Assessing communication competence in an online study: Toward informing subsequent interventions among older adults with cancer, their lay caregivers, and peers. *Health Communication*, 15: 203–18.

Rabow, M., Hauser, J., and Adams, J. (2004). The role of nurse practitioners in end-of-life care. *Journal of the American Medical Association*, 291: 483–91.

Radina, M. E., Gibbons, H. M., and Lim, J. (2009). Explicit versus implicit family decision-making strategies among Mexican American caregiving adult children. *Marriage and Family Review*, 45: 392–411.

Ragan, M. (2010, January 7). *Facebook: OSU Shares Timely Health Info* [Web log message]. Retrieved from: <http://www.prdaily.com/ME2/Sites/Default.asp?SiteID=5F41200A5 35341AD8E013330C55EA38D>.

Ragan, S. L., and Glenn, L. D. (1990). Communication and gynecologic health care. In H. D. O'Hair and G. Kreps (eds), *Applied Communication Theory and Research* (pp. 313–30). Hillsdale, NJ: Erlbaum.

Ragan, S. L., and Goldsmith, J. (2008). End-of-life communication: The drama of pretense in the talk of dying patients and their M.D.s. In K. B. Wright and S. C. Moore (eds), *Applied Health Communication: A Sourcebook* (pp. 207–27). Boston, MA: Allyn and Bacon.

Ragan, S. L., Wittenberg, E., and Hall, H. T. (2003). The communication of palliative care for the elderly cancer patient. *Health Communication*, 15: 219–26.

Ragan, S. L., Wittenberg-Lyles, E. M., Goldsmith, J. and Sanchez-Reilly, S. (2008). Communicating a terminal prognosis in a palliative care setting: Deficiencies in current communication training protocols. *Social Science and Medicine*, 66: 2356–65.

Rains, Stephen A. (2008). Seeking health information in the information age: the role of Internet self-efficacy. *Western Journal of Communication*, 72: 1–19.

Rait, D., and Lederberg, M. (1989). The family of the cancer patient. In J. C. Holland, and J. H. Rowland (eds), *Handbook of Psychooncology: Psychological Care of the Patient with Cancer* (pp. 585–97). Oxford University Press: New York.

Raman, P., et al. (2004, June). *Older Adult Portrayals in Indian and US Magazine Advertisements*. Paper presented at the Ninth International Conference on Language and Social Psychology, State College, PA.

Ramanadhan, S., and Viswanath, K. (2006). Health and the information nonseeker: A profile. *Health Communication*, 20(2): 131–9.

Ramirez, A. G. (2003). Consumer–provider communication research with special populations. *Patient Education and Counseling*, 50: 51–4.

Ramsay, J. O., and Silverman, B. W. (2002). *Applied Functional Data Analysis: Methods and Case Studies*. New York, NY: Springer-Verlag.

Ramsay, S. (1999). International research agenda set for end-of-life care. *Lancet*, 354: 1361.

Raphael, C., Ahrens, J., and Fowler, N. (2001). Financing end-of-life care in the USA. *Journal of the Royal Society of Medicine*, 94: 458–61.

Rappaport, J. (1993). Narrative studies, personal stories, and identity transformation in the mutual help context. *Journal of Applied Behavioral Science*, 29: 239–56.

Ratner, E., Norlander, L., and McSteen, K. (2001). Death at home following a targeted advanced-care planning process at home: The kitchen table discussion. *Journal of the American Geriatrics Society*, 49: 778–81.

Ratzan, S. (ed.). (1994). Health communication: Challenges for the 21st century. *American Behavioral Scientist*, 38(2): 197–380.

Ratzan, S. C., et al. (2000). Attaining global health: challenges and opportunities. *Population Bulletin*, 55: 3–48.

Rayburn, T. M., and Stonecypher, J. F. (1996). Diagnostic differences related to age and race of involuntarily committed psychiatric patients. *Psychological Reports*, 79: 881–2.

Rea, M. (2010, January 4). *What Goes On Outside the Exam Room Can Have a Big Impact on Your Practice* [Web log message]. Retrieved from: <http://www.articlesbase.com/marketing-tips-articles/what-goes-on-outside-the-exam-room-can-have-a-big-impact-on-your-practice-1666134.html>.

Reb, A. M. (2003). Palliative and end-of-life care: Policy analysis. *Oncology Nursing Forum*, 30: 35–50.

Reicher, S. (1986). Contact, action and racialization: Some British evidence. In M. Hewstone and R. Brown (eds), *Contact and Conflict in Intergroup Encounters* (pp. 152–68). Cambridge, MA: Blackwell.

Reicher, S. D. (1987). Crowd behavior as social action. In J. C. Turner, et al. (eds), *Rediscovering the Social Group: A Self-categorization Theory* (pp. 171–202). Oxford: Blackwell.

Reid, S., and Giles, H. (2005). Intergroup relations: Its linguistic and communicative parameters. *Group Processes and Intergroup Relations*, 8: 211–14.

Repetto, L., Piselli, P., Raffaele, M., and Locatelli, C. (2009). Communicating cancer diagnosis and prognosis: When the target is the elderly patient. *European Journal of Cancer*, 45: 374–83.

Rhymes, J. (1990). Hospice care in America. *Journal of the American Medical Association*, 264: 369.

Rice, R. E., and Katz, J. E. (eds). (2001). *The Internet and Health Communication: Experiences and Expectations*. Thousand Oaks, CA: Sage Publications.

Richards, L. Bengston, V., and Miller, R. (1989). The "generation in the middle": Perceptions of changes in adult intergenerational relationships. In K. Kreppner and R. Lerner (eds), *Family Systems and Life Span Development* (pp. 341–66). Hillsdale, NJ: Erlbaum.

Richey, J. A. (2003). *Women in Alaska Constructing the Recovered Self: A Narrative Approach to Understanding Long-term Recovery from Alcohol Dependence and/or Abuse.* [Doctoral dissertation, University of Alaska Fairbanks]. Retrieved from: <http://proquest.umi.com>.

Riessman, F. (1965). The "helper" therapy principle. *Social Work*, 10: 27–32.

Rimal, R., and Adkins, A. (2003). Using computers to narrowcast health messages: The role of audience segmentation, targeting, and tailoring in health promotion. In T. Thompson, A. Dorsey, K. Miller, and R. Parrott (eds), *Handbook of Health Communication* (pp. 497–513). Mahwah, NJ: Lawrence Erlbaum.

Rivadeneyra, R., Elderkin-Thompson, V., Cohen-Silver, R., and Waitzkin, H. (2000). Patient-centeredness in medical encounters requiring an interpreter. *American Journal of Medicine*, 108: 470–4.

Rob. (2009, November 17). *Bad News in Being a Doctor* [Web log message]. Retrieved from: <http://distractible.org/2009/11/17/bad-news/>.

Roberts, C. S., and Cox, C. F. (1997). Medical and psychosocial treatment issues in breast cancer in older women. *Journal of Gerontological Social Work*, 28: 63–74.

Robin, M. (1999). Explanations of ethnic and gender differences in youth smoking: A multi-site, qualitative investigation. *Nicotine and Tobacco Research*, 1: S91–S98.

Robinson, J. D. (1998). Getting down to business: Talk, gaze, and body orientation during openings of doctor–patient consultations. *Human Communication Research*, 25: 97–123.

Robinson, J. D., and Heritage, J. (2005). The structure of patients' presenting concerns: the completion relevance of current symptoms. *Social Science and Medicine*, 61: 481–93.

Robinson, J. D., and Heritage, J. (2006). Physicians' opening questions and patients' satisfaction. *Patient Education and Counseling*, 60: 279–85.

Rodriguez, M. M., Casper, G. and Brennan, P. F. (2007). Patient-centered design: The potential of user-centered design in personal health records. *Journal of AHIMA*, 78(4): 44–6.

Rogers, E. M. (1995). *Diffusion of Innovations* (4th edn). New York: Free Press.

Rogers, E. M. (2003). *Diffusion of Innovations* (5th edn). New York: Free Press.

Rogers, E. M. (2004). A prospective and retrospective look at the diffusion model. *Journal of Health Communication*, 9: 13–20.

Rogers, R. W. (1975). A protection motivation theory of fear appeals and attitude change. *Journal of Psychology*, 91: 93–114.

Rogers, R. W. (1983). Cognitive and physiological processes in fear appeals and attitude change: A revised theory of protection motivation. In J. Cacioppo and R. Petty (eds), *Social Psychophysiology* (pp. 153–76). New York: Guilford.

Rook, K. (1995). Support, companionship, and control in older adults' social networks: Implications for well-being. In J. F. Nussbaum and J. Coupland (eds), *Handbook of Communication and Aging Research* (pp. 437–63). Mahwah, NJ: Lawrence Erlbaum Associates.

Roschelle, A. R. (1997). *No More Kin: Exploring Race, Class, and Gender in Family Networks.* Thousand Oaks, CA: Sage.

Rose, J. H., Bowman, K., and Kresevic, D. (2000). Nurse versus family caregiver perspectives on hospitalized older patients: An exploratory study of agreement at admission and discharge. *Health Communication*, 12: 63–80.

Rosenberg, P. P. (1984). Support groups: A special therapeutic entity. *Small Group Behavior*, 15: 173–86.

Rosenberg, E., Richard, C., Lussier, M. T., and Abdool, S. N. (2006). Intercultural communication competence in family medicine: Lessons from the field. *Patient Education and Counseling*, 61(2): 236–45.

Rosenstock, I. M. (1974). Historical origins of the health belief model. *Health Education Monographs*, 2: 328–35.

Ross, C. E., Mirowski, J., and Cockerham, W. C. (1983). Social class, Mexican culture, and fatalism: their effects on psychological distress. *American Journal of Community Psychology*, 11: 383–99.

Ross, S. E., et al. (2005). Expectations of Patients and Physicians Regarding Patient-Accessible Medical Records, *Journal of Medical Internet Research*, 7: e13.

Roter, D. L., and Hall, J. A. (1993): *Doctors Talking with Patients/Patients Talking with Doctors*. Westport, CT: Auburn House.

Roter, D. L., Hall, J. A. and Aoki, Y. (2002) Physician gender effects in medical communication: A meta-analytic review. *Journal of the American Medical Association*, 288: 756–64.

Roter, D. L., et al. (1995). Improving physicians' interviewing skills and reducing patients' emotional distress. *Archives of Internal Medicine*, 9: 222–6.

Roter, D. L., et al. (1997). Communication patterns of primary care physicians. *The Journal of the American Medical Association*, 277: 350–6.

Rothchild, E. (1994). Family dynamics in end-of-life treatment decisions. *General Hospital Psychiatry*, 16: 251–8.

Rothman, A. J., et al. (1993). The influence of message framing on intentions to perform health behaviors. *Journal of Experimental Social Psychology*, 29(5): 408.

Rowan, K. (2008). Monthly communication skills training for healthcare staff, *Patient Education and Counseling*, 71: 402–4.

Rucker-Whitaker, C., Feinglass, J., and Pearce, W. H. (2003). Explaining racial variation in lower extremity amputation. *Archives of Surgery*, 138: 1347–51.

Rudd, R. (2007). Health literacy skills of U. S. adults. *American Journal of Health Behavior*, 31: S8–S18.

Ruscher, J. (2001). *Prejudiced Communication*. New York: Guilford Press.

Rusinak, R. L., and Murphy, J. F. (1995). Elderly spousal caregivers: Knowledge of cancer care, perceptions of preparedness, and coping strategies. *Journal of Gerontological Nursing*, 21: 33–41.

Rutten, L. F., and Arora, N. (2007). Importance of physicians' communication behavior across the cancer care continuum. In D. O'Hair, G. Kreps, and L. Sparks (eds), *Handbook of Communication and Cancer Care* (pp. 13–35). Creskill, NJ: Hampton Press.

Rutten, L. J. F., Squiers, L., and Hesse, B. (2006). Cancer-related information seeking: Hints from the 2003 Health Information National Trends Survey (HINTS). *Journal of Health Communication*, 11(s1): 147–56.

Ryan, E. B., Meredith, S. D., MacLean, M. J., and Orange, J. B. (1995). Changing the way we talk with elders: Promoting health using the communication enhancement model. *International Journal of Aging and Human Development*, 41: 89–107.

Sabogal, F., et al. (1987). Hispanic familiasm and acculturation: What changes and what doesn't? *Hispanic Journal of Behavioral Sciences*, 4: 397–412.

Sack, K., and Kolata, G. (2009, November 18). Screening policy won't change, U.S. officials say. *The New York Times*. Retrieved from: <http://www.nytimes.com/2009/11/19/health/19cancer.html?emc=eta1>.

Safeer, R. S., and Keenan, J. (2005). Health literacy: The gap between physicians and patients. *American Family Physician*, 72: 463.

Sahlstein, E. M. (2004). Relating at a distance: Negotiating being together and being apart in long-distance relationships. *Journal of Social and Personal Relationships*, 21: 689–710.

Sahlstein, E. M. (2006a). Making plans: Praxis strategies for negotiating uncertainty-certainty in long-distance relationships. *Western Journal of Communication,* 70: 147–65.

Sahlstein, E. M. (2006b). The trouble with distance. In D. C. Kirkpatrick, S. Duck, and M. K. Foley (eds), *Relating Difficulty: The Processes of Constructing and Managing Difficult Interaction* (pp. 119–40). Mahwah, NJ: Erlbaum.

Saks, E. R. (2009). Some thoughts on denial of mental illness. *American Journal of Psychiatry,* 166: 972–3.

Sala, F., Krupat, E., and Roter, D. (2002). Satisfaction and the use of humor by physicians and patients. *Health and Psychology,* 17: 269–80.

Sandman, P. M. (1993). *Responding to Community Outrage: Strategies for Effective Risk Communication.* Fairfax, VA: American Industrial Hygiene Association.

Sarason, B. R., Sarason, I. G., and Garung, R. A. F. (1997). Close personal relationships and health outcomes: A key to the role of social support. In S. Duck (ed.), *Handbook of Personal Relationships* (2nd edn, pp. 547–73). New York: Wiley.

Sarason, B. R., Sarason, I. G. and Pierce, G. R. (1990). *Social Support: An Interactional View.* New York, NY: Wiley.

Sarna, L., and Brecht, M. (1997). Dimensions of symptom distress in women with advanced lung cancer: A factor analysis. *Heart and Lung,* 26: 23–30.

Sarna, L., and McCorkle, R. (1996). Burden of care and lung cancer. *Cancer Practice,* 4: 245–51.

Sass, J. S. (2000). Emotional labor as cultural performance: The communication of caregiving in a nonprofit nursing home. *Western Journal of Communication,* 64(3): 330–58.

Scanzoni, J., and Polonko, K. (1980). A conceptual approach to explicit marital negotiation. *Journal of Marriage and the Family,* 42: 31–44.

Schein, E. H. (1985). *Organizational Culture and Leadership.* San Francisco, CA: Jossey-Bass.

Schillinger, D., et al. (2006). Does literacy mediate the relationship between education and health outcomes?: A study of a low income population with diabetes. *Public Health Reports,* 121: 245–54.

Schimmel, S. R. (1999). *Cancer Talk: Voices of Hope and Endurance from "The Group Room," the World's Largest Cancer Support Group.* New York: Broadway Books.

Scholl, J. (2007). The use of humor to promote patient-centered care. *Journal of Applied Communication Research,* 35(2):156–76.

Scholl, J., and Ragan, S. (2003). The use of humor in promoting positive provider–patient interactions in a hospital rehabilitation unit. *Health Communication,* 15: 319–30.

Schoonover, C. B., Brody, E. M., Hoffman, C., and Kleban, M. H. (1988). Parent care and geographically distant children. *Research on Aging,* 10: 472–92.

Segrin, C. (2003). Age moderates the relationship between social support and psychosocial problems. *Human Communication Research,* 29: 317–42.

Seijo, R., Gomez, H., and Freidenberg, J. (1991). Language as a communication barrier in medical care for Hispanic patients. *Hispanic Journal of Behavioral Science,* 13: 363–73.

Sellnow, T. L., Seeger, M. W., and Ulmer, R. R. (2003). Chaos theory, informational needs, and natural disasters. *Journal of Applied Communication Research,* 30(4): 269–92.

Senak, M. (2009, December 16). *Pharma and YouTube – Where are the Eyeballs Going?* [Web log message]. Retrieved from: <http://www.eyeonfda.com/eye_on_fda/2009/12/pharma-and-youtube-where-are-the-eyeballs-going.html#comments>.

Sentell, T., and Halpin, H. A. (2006). The importance of adult literacy in understanding health disparities. *Journal of General Internal Medicine,* 21: 862–6.

Shapiro, J., and Saltzer, E. (1981). Cross-cultural aspects of physician–patient communication patterns. *Urban Health,* 10(10): 10–15.

Sharf, B. F., and Street, R. L. (1997). The patient as a central construct: Shifting the emphasis. *Health Communication*, 9(1): 1–11.

Sheehy, E., et al. (2003). Estimating the number of potential organ donors in the United States. *The New England Journal of Medicine*, 349: 667–74.

Sheeran, P., and Abraham, C. (1996). The health belief model. In M. Conner and P. Norman (eds), *Predicting Health Behaviour: Research and Practice with Social Cognition Models* (pp. 23–61). Bristol, PA: The Open University.

Shin, B. H., and Bruno, R. (2003) Language use and English speaking ability: Census 2000 brief. *US Census Bureau*. Retrieved from: <http://www.census.gov/prod/2003pubs/c2kbr-29.pdf>.

Shinnar, R. (2008). Coping with negative social identity: The case of Mexican immigrants. *The Journal of Social Psychology*, 148: 553–75.

Siegel, K., Raveis, V. H., Houts, P., and Mor, V. (1991). Caregiver burden and unmet patient needs. *Cancer*, 68: 1131–40.

Sillars, A., Roberts, L. J., Leonard, K. E., and Dun, T. (2000). Cognition during marital conflict: The relationship of thought and talk. *Journal of Social and Personal Relationships*, 17: 479–502.

Sillars, A. L. (1980). Attributions and communication in roommate conflicts. *Communication Monographs*, 47: 180–200.

Siminoff, L. A., Ravdin, P., Colabianchi, N., and Sturm, C. M. S. (2000). Doctor–patient communication patterns in breast cancer adjuvant therapy discussions. *Health Expectations*, 3: 26–36.

Sleath, B., and Rubin, R. H. (2002). Gender, ethnicity, and physician–patient communication about depression and anxiety in primary care. *Patient Education and Counseling*, 48: 243–52.

Sleath, B., Rubin, R. H., and Wurst, K. (2003). The influence of Hispanic ethnicity on patients' expressions of complaints about and problems with adherence to antidepressant therapy. *Clinical Therapeutics*, 25: 1739–49.

Smedley, B. D., Stith, A. Y., and Nelson, A. R.. (2003). *Unequal Treatment: Confronting Racial and Ethnic Disparities in Health Care*. Washington, DC: National Academics Press.

Smith, E. (2009, September 19). Medical interpreters break language barriers in health care. *Medical News Today*. Retrieved from: <http://www.medicalnewstoday.com/articles/164444.php>.

Smith, G. C. (1998). Residential separation and patterns of interaction between elderly parents and their adult children. *Progress in Human Geography*, 22: 368–84.

Smith, R. A., Cokkinides, V., and Brawley, O. W. (2009). Cancer screening in the United States, 2009: A review of current American Cancer Society guidelines and issues in cancer screening. *CA: Cancer Journal for Clinicians*, 59: 27–41.

Smith, V. L. (2009, October 16). The ABC dilemma of health reform. *The Wall Street Journal*. Retrieved from: <http://online.wsj.com/article/SB100014240527487032980045744553037298263632.html>.

Smith duPré, A., and Beck, C. S. (1996). Enabling patients and physicians to pursue multiple goals in health care encounters: A case study. *Health Communication*, 8: 73–90.

Solis, B. (2007, February 19). *What's Wrong with Social Media?* [Web log message]. Retrieved from: <http://www.briansolis.com/2007/02/whats-wrong-with-social-media/>.

Soliz, J. (2004). Shared family identity, age salience, and intergroup contact: Investigation of the grandparent–grandchild relationship. Unpublished dissertation: University of Kansas.

Sparks, L. (2003a). An introduction to cancer communication and aging: Theoretical and research insights. *Health Communication*, 15: 123–32.

Sparks, L. (ed.). (2003b). Cancer communication and aging [Special Issue]. *Health Communication*, 15(2): 123–258.

Sparks, L. (2007). Cancer care and the aging patient: Complexities of age–related communication barriers. In H. D. O'Hair, L. Sparks, and G. L. Kreps (eds), *Handbook of Communication and Cancer Care* (pp. 233–49). Cresskill, NJ: Hampton Press.

Sparks, L. (2008). Family decision-making. In W. Donsbach (ed.) The *International Encyclopedia of Communication*, 4, (pp. 1729–33). Oxford, UK and Malden, MA: Wiley-Blackwell.

Sparks, L. (forthcoming). Health communication and caregiving research, policy, and practice. In R. Talley (ed.) *Caregiving across the Professions*. New York: Springer.

Sparks, L., and Harwood, J. (2008). Cancer, aging, and social identity: Development of an integrated model of social identity theory and health communication. In L. Sparks, H. D. O'Hair, and G. L. Kreps, (eds), *Cancer Communication and Aging* (pp. 77–95). Cresskill, NJ: Hampton Press.

Sparks, L., and Hill, L. B. (2005). Personal relationships across the lifespan: A suggestive perspective from communication theory. *Intercultural Communication Studies*, XIV: 158–71.

Sparks, L., and McPherson, J. (2007). Cross-cultural differences in choices of health information by older cancer patients and their family caregivers. In K. B. Wright and S. D. Moore (eds), *Applied Health Communication* (pp. 179–205). Cresskill, NJ: Hampton Press.

Sparks, L., and Mittapalli, K. (2004). To know or not to know: The case of communication by and with older adult Russians diagnosed with cancer. *Journal of Cross Cultural Gerontology*, 19: 383–403.

Sparks, L. and Nussbaum, J. F. (2008). Health literacy and cancer communication with older adults. *Patient Education and Counseling*, 71(3): 345–50.

Sparks, L., and Turner, M. M. (2008). Cognitive and emotional processing of cancer messages and information seeking with older adults. In L. Sparks, H. D. O'Hair, and G. L. Kreps, (eds), *Cancer Communication and Aging* (pp. 17–45). Cresskill, NJ: Hampton Press.

Sparks, L., and Villagran, M. (2008). *La Comunicación en el Cancer: Comunicación y apoyo emocional en el laberinto del cancer.* [English translation: *Communication and Emotional Support in the Cancer Maze.*] Spain: Aresta

Sparks, L., and Villagran, M. M. (2009). *Talking Cancer*. Spain: Aresta.

Sparks, L., O'Hair, H. D., and Kreps, G. L. (eds). (2008a). *Cancer Communication and Aging*. Cresskill, NJ: Hampton Press.

Sparks, L., O'Hair, H. D. and Kreps, G. L. (2008b). Conceptualizing cancer communication and aging: New directions for research. In L. Sparks, H. D. O'Hair, and G. L. Kreps, (eds), *Cancer Communication and Aging* (pp. 1–14). Cresskill, NJ: Hampton Press.

Sparks, L., Travis, S., and Thompson, S. (2005). Listening for the communicative signals of humor, narratives, and self-disclosure in the family caregiving interview. *Health and Social Work*, 30: 340–3.

Sparks, L., Villagran, M., Parker-Raley, J., and Cunningham, C. (2007). A patient-centered approach to breaking bad news: Communication guidelines for health care providers. *Journal of Applied Communication Research*, 35; 177–96.

Sparks-Bethea, L. (2001). The function of humor within the lives of older adults. *Qualitative Research Reports in Communication*, 2: 49–56.

Sparks-Bethea, L. (2002). The impact of an older adult parent on communicative satisfaction and dyadic adjustment in the long-term marital relationship: Adult children and spouses' retrospective accounts. *Journal of Applied Communication Research*, 30: 107–25.

Sparks-Bethea, L. and Balazs, A. (1997). Improving intergenerational healthcare communication. *Journal of Health Communication*, 2: 129–37.

Sparks-Bethea, L., Travis, S. S., and Pecchioni, L. L. (2000). Family caregivers' use of humor in conveying information about caring for dependent older adults. *Health Communication*, 12: 361–76.

Spiegel, D. (1992). Effects of psychosocial support on patients with metastatic breast cancer. *Journal of Psychosocial Oncology*, 10: 113–21.

Spiegel, D., and Bloom, J. R. (1983). Pain in metastatic breast cancer. *Cancer*, 52: 149–53.

Spiegel, D., Bloom, J. R., and Yalom, I. (1981). Group support for patients with metastatic cancer: A randomized prospective outcome study. *Archives of General Psychiatry*, 38: 527–33.

Squiers, L., et al. (2005). Cancer patients' information needs across the cancer care continuum: Evidence from the Cancer Information Service. *Journal of Health Communication*, 10(s1): 15–34.

Stafford, L. (2005). Maintaining long-distance and cross-residential relationships. Mahwah, NJ: Erlbaum.

Steinhart, B. (2002). Patient autonomy: evolution of the doctor–patient relationship. *Haemophilia*, 8: 441–6.

Stewart, M., and Brown, J. B. (2001). Towards a global definition of patient centered care. *British Medical Journal*, 322: 444–5.

Stewart, M., et al. (2000). The impact of patient-centered care on outcomes. *Journal of Family Practice*, 49: 796–804.

Stohl, C., and Cheney, G. (2001). Participatory processes/paradoxical practices: Communication and the dilemmas of organizational democracy. *Management Communication Quarterly*, 14: 349–407.

Stoller, E. P., Forster, L. E., Duniho, D. S. (1992). Systems of parent care within sibling networks. *Research on Aging*, 14: 28–49.

Stoltz, P., Uden, G., and Willman, A. (2004). Support for family carers who care for an elderly person at home – a systematic literature review. *Scandinavian Journal of Caring Sciences*, 18: 111–19.

Stott, C., and Reicher, S. (1998). Crowd action as intergroup process: Introducing the police perspective. *European Journal of Social Psychology*, 28: 509–29.

Street, A., and Blackford, J. (2001). Communication issues for the interdisciplinary community palliative care team. *Journal of Clinical Nursing*, 10: 643–50.

Street, R. L. Jr. (2001). Active patients as powerful communicators. In W. P. Robinson and H. Giles (eds), *The New Handbook of Language and Social Psychology*, (pp. 541–60), Chichester, UK: John Wiley.

Street, R. L. (2007). Aiding medical decision-making: A communication perspective. *Medical Decision-making*, 10: 550–3.

Street, R. L., Jr, and Gordon, H. (2008). Companion participation in cancer consultations. *Psycho-Oncology*, 17: 244–51.

Street, R. L., Jr., Gordon, H. S., and Haidet, P. (2007). Physicians' communication and perceptions of patients: Is it how they look, how they talk, or is it just the doctor? *Social Science and Medicine*, 65: 586–98.

Street, R. L., et al. (2003). Beliefs about control in the physician–patient relationship: Effect on communication in medical encounters. *The Journal of General Internal Medicine*, 18: 609–16.

Street, R. L., et al. (2005). Patient participation in medical consultations: Why some patients are more involved than others. *Medical Care*, 43: 960–9.

Street, R. L. Jr. O'Malley, K. J., Cooper, L. A., and Haidet, P. (2008). Understanding concordance in patient–physician relationships: Personal and ethnic dimensions of shared identity. *Annals of Family Medicine*, 6: 1–22.

Stroman, C. (2000). Explaining illness to African Americans: Employing cultural concerns with strategies. In B. Whaley (ed.), *Explaining Illness: Research, Theory, and Strategies* (pp. 299–316). Mahwah, NJ: Lawrence Erlbaum.

Stryker, S. (1987). Identity theory: Developments and extensions. In K. Hardley and T. Honess (eds). *Self and Identity* (pp. 89–104). New York: Wiley.

Suchman, A., Markakis, K., Beckman, H. B., and Frankel, R. (1997). A model of empathic communication in the medical interview. *Journal of the American Medical Association*, 277: 678–82.

Suler, J. R. (2004). The online disinhibition effect. *CyberPsychology and Behavior*, 7: 321–6.

Sullivan, C. F., and Reardon, K. K. (1985). Social support satisfaction and health locus of control: Discriminators of breast cancer patients' style of coping. In M. L. McLaughlin (ed.), *Communication Yearbook* (Vol. 9, pp. 707–22). Beverly Hills, CA: Sage.

Swenson, S. L., et al. (2004). Patient-centered communication: Do patients really prefer it?. *Journal of General Internal Medicine*, 19: 1069–79.

Sykes, N. (1989). Medical students' fears about breaking bad news. *Lancet*, 2: 564.

Tait, P. (2007). *The Doctor's Communication Handbook*. Oxford: Radcliffe.

Tajfel, H., and Turner, J. C. (1986). The social identity theory of intergroup behavior. In S. Worschel and W. G. Austin (eds), *The Social Psychology of Intergroup Relations* (2nd edn, pp. 7–24). Chicago, IL: Nelson-Hall.

Takayama, T., Yamazaki, Y., and Katsumata, N. (2001). Relationship between outpatients' perceptions of physicians' communication styles and patients' anxiety levels in a Japanese oncology setting. *Social Science and Medicine*, 53(10): 1335–50.

Talamantes, M. A., Gomez, C., and Braun, K. L. (2000). Advance directives and end-of-life care: The Hispanic perspective. In K. L. Braun, J. H. Pietsch, and P. L. Blanchette (eds), *Cultural Issues in End-of-Life Decision Making* (pp. 83–100). Thousand Oaks, CA: Sage.

Tamayo, G. J., Broxson, A., Munsell, M., and Cohen, M. Z. (2010). Caring for the caregiver. *Oncology Nursing Forum*, 37: E50–E57.

Teno, J. M., et al. (2004). Family perspectives on end-of-life care at the last place of care. *Journal of the American Medical Association*, 291(1): 88–93.

Teslik, L. H., and Johnson, T. (2009). Healthcare costs and U.S. competitiveness. *Council of Foreign Relations*. Retrieved from: <http://www.cfr.org/publication/13325/>.

Thois, P. A. (1991). On merging identity theory and stress research. *Social Psychological Quarterly*, 54: 101–12.

Thoits, P. (1982). Conceptual, methodological, and theoretical problems in studying social support as a buffer against life stress. *Journal of Health and Social Behavior*, 23: 145–59.

Thomas, S. B., Fine, M. J., and Ibrahim, S. A. (2004). Health disparities: The importance of culture and health. *American Journal of Public Health*, 94: 9–36.

Thompson, S. C., Armstrong, W., and Thomas, C. (1998). Illusions of control, underestimation, and accuracy: A control psychological explanation. *Psychological Bulletin*, 123: 143–61.

Thompson, T. L. (1984). The invisible helping hand: The role of communication in the health and social service professions. *Communication Quarterly*, 32(2): 148–63.

Thompson, T. L. (2000). The nature and language of illness explanations. In B. B. Whaley (ed.), *Explaining Illness: Research, Theory, and Strategies* (pp. 3–40). Mahwah, NJ: Erlbaum.

Thompson, T. L., Dorsey, A. M., Miller, K. I., and Parrott, R. (eds). (2003). *Handbook of Health Communication*. Mahwah, NJ: Lawrence Erlbaum.

Thoresen, C. E., and Harris, A. H. S. (2002). Spirituality and health: What's the evidence and what's needed? *Annals of Behavioral Medicine*, 24: 3–13.

Thornley, J. (2008, April 8). *What is 'Social Media?'* [Web log message]. Retrieved from: <http://propr.ca/2008/what-is-social-media/>.

Ting-Toomey, S. (1999). *Communicating across Cultures*. New York: Guilford.

Tinley, S., et al. (2004). Screening adherence in BRCA1/2 families is associated with primary physician's behavior. *American Journal of Medical Genetics*, 125(1): 5–11.

Todorov, A., Chaiken, S. and Henderson, M. D. (2002). The heuristic-systematic model of social information processing. In J. P. Dillard, and M. Pfau (eds), *The Persuasion Handbook: Developments in Theory and Practice* (pp. 195–212). Thousand Oaks, CA: Sage Publications.

Tompkins, P. and Cheney, G. (1985). Communication and unobtrusive control in contemporary organizations. In R. D. McPhee and P. K. Thompkins (eds), *Organizational Communication: Traditional Themes and New Directions* (pp. 179–210). Beverly Hills, CA: Sage.

Toseland, R. W., Blanchard, C. G., and McCallion, P. (1995). A problem solving intervention for caregivers of cancer patients. *Social Science in Medicine*, 40: 517–28.

Towers Perrin. (2008). *Update on U.S. Tort Cost Trends*. Retrieved from: <http://www.towersperrin.com/tp/getwebcachedoc?webc=USA/2008/200811/2008_tort_costs_trends.pdf>.

Trapp, R., and Hoff, N. (1985). A model of serial argument in interpersonal relationships. *Journal of the American Forensic Association*, 22: 1–11.

Travis, S. S., and Piercy, K. (2002). Family caregivers. In I. Lubkin and P. Larsen (eds) (5th edn). *Chronic Illness: Impact and Interventions* (pp. 233–60). Sudbury, MA: Jones and Bartlett Publishers.

Travis, S. S., and Sparks-Bethea, L. (2001). Medication administration by family members of dependent elders in shared care arrangements. *Journal of Clinical Geropsychology*, 7(3): 231–43.

Travis, S., Sparks-Bethea, L., and Winn, P. (2000). Medication hassles reported by family caregivers of dependent elders. *Journals of Gerontology: Medical Sciences*, 55A: 7, M412–M417.

Triandis, H. C. (1995). *Individualism and Collectivism*. Boulder, CO: Westview.

Tu, H. T., and Lauer, J. (2008). *Word of Mouth and Physician Referrals Still Drive Health Care Provider Choice* (Research Brief No. 9). Retrieved from Center for Studying Health System Change website: <http://www.hschange.org/CONTENT/1028/>.

Tulsky, J. A. (2005). Beyond advance directives: Importance of communication skills at the end of life. *Journal of the American Medical Association*, 294: 359–65.

Turner, J. C. et al. (1987). *Rediscovering the social group: A Self-categorization Theory.* Cambridge, MA: Blackwell.

Turner, J. W. (2003). Telemedicine: Expanding healthcare into virtual environments. In T. L. Thompson, A. M. Dorsey, K. I. Miller, and R. Parrott (eds), *Handbook of Health Communication* (pp. 515–35). Mahwah, NJ: Lawrence Erlbaum.

Turner, R. A., King, P. R., and Tremblay, P. F. (1992). Coping styles and depression among psychiatric outpatients. *Personality and Individual Differences*, 13: 1145–7.

Turner, T., et al. (2009). Pediatricians and health literacy: Descriptive results from a national survey. *Pediatrics*, 124: S299–S305.

Tversky, A., and Kahneman, D. (1981). The framing of decisions and the psychology of choice. *Science*, 211: 453–8.

Uchino, B. N., Cacioppo, J. T., and Kiecolt-Glaser, J. K. (1996). The relationship between social support and physiological processes: A review with emphasis on underlying mechanisms and implications for health. *Psychological Bulletin*, 119: 488–531.

Ulene, V. (2009, March 9). Bad news, bad delivery. *Los Angeles Times*, p. E3.

Uncapher, H., and Arean, P. A. (2000). Physicians are less willing to treat suicidal ideation in older patients. *Journal of the American Geriatrics Society*, 48(2): 188–92.

United Network For Organ Sharing (2008). *Annual Report Data*. Retrieved from: <http://unos.org/data/about/viewDataReports.asp>.

US Census Bureau. (2003). *Language Use and English-speaking Ability: 2000*. Washington, DC: US Census Bureau.

US Department of Education, National Center for Education Statistics, Institute of Education Sciences, National Assessment of Adult Literacy (2007). *Literacy in Everday*

Life: Results from the 2003 National Assessment of Adult Literacy (NCES Publication No. 2007-480). Retrieved from: <http://nces.ed.gov/Pubs2007/2007480.pdf>.

US Department of Health and Human Services. (2000). *Healthy people 2010*. Atlanta, GA: CDC. Retrieved September 30, 2005. Available at: <http://www.healthypeople.gov/>.

US Department of Health and Human Services. (2010). *Quick Guide to Health Literacy*. Retrieved from: <http://www.health.gov/communication/literacy/quickguide/about.htm>.

Van Knippenberg, D. (1999). Social identity and persuasion: Reconsidering the role of group membership. In D. Abrams and M. A. Hogg (eds), *Social Identity and Social Cognition* (pp. 315–31). Malden, MA: Blackwell.

Van Servellen, G. (2009). *Communication Skills for the Health Care Professional: Concepts, Practice, and Evidence* (2nd edn). Sudbury, MA: Jones and Bartlett.

Van Straten, A., Cuijpers, P. and Smits, N. (2008). Effectiveness of a Web-based self-help intervention for symptoms of depression, anxiety, and stress: Randomized controlled trial. *Journal of Medical Internet Research*, 10(1): e7.

Van Winkle, N. W. (2000). End-of-life decision making in American Indian and Alaska Native cultures. In K. L. Braun, J. H. Pietsch, and P. L. Blanchette (eds), *Cultural Issues in End-of-Life Decision Making* (pp. 127–44). Thousand Oaks, CA: Sage.

Vanderford, M., Jenks, E., and Sharf, B. (1997). Exploring patients' experiences as a primary source of meaning. *Health Communication*, 9(1): 13–26.

Vanlandingham, M. J., Suprasert, S., Grandjean, N., and Sittitrai, W. (1995). Two views of risky sexual practices among northern Thai males: The health belief model and the theory of reasoned action. *Journal of Health and Social Behavior*, 36: 195–212.

Villagran, M., and Hoffman (2008). Creating culturally appropriate organizational communication messages to combat health disparities in cancer care. In L. Sparks, H. D. O'Hair, and G. L. Kreps, (eds), *Cancer Communication and Aging* (pp. 259–75). Cresskill, NJ: Hampton Press.

Villagran, M. M., and Hoffman, M. F. (2009). Knowledge is *still* power. In J. Keyton and P. Shockley-Zalabak (eds) *Case Studies for Organizational Communication: Understanding Processes* (3rd edn, pp. 73–75). Los Angeles, CA: Roxbury Press.

Villagran, M., and Lucke, J. (2005). Translating communication measures for use with non-English-speaking populations. *Communication Research Reports*, 22: 247–51.

Villagran, M. M., and Sparks, L. (2010). Social identity in the patient–provider interaction. In J. Harwood, H. Giles, and S. Reid (eds), *The Dynamics of Intergroup Communication* (pp. 235–48). New York: Peter Lang.

Villagran, M., Collins, D., and Garcia, S. (2008) Voces de Las Colonias: Dialectical Tensions about Control and Cultural Identification in Latinas' Communication about Cancer. In H. Zoller and M. Dutta (eds), *Emerging Issues and Perspectives in Health Communication: Meaning, Culture, Power* (pp. 203–23). New York: Routledge.

Villagran, M., Fox, L., and O'Hair, H. D. (2007). Patient communication processes: Agency, identity, and cancer care. In H. D. O'Hair, L. Sparks, and G. L. Kreps (eds), *Handbook of Communication and Cancer Care* (pp. 131–48). Cresskill, NJ: Hampton Press.

Villagran, M., Wittenberg-Lyles, E., and Hajek, C. (2007, November). *The Impact of Communication, Attitudes, and Acculturation on Advance Directives Decision-making*. Paper presented at the Annual Convention, Chicago. Retrieved from: <http://www.allacademic.com/meta/p194018_index.html>.

Villagran, M. M., Weathers, M., Keefe, B., and Sparks, L. (2010). Medical providers as global warming and climate change health educators: A health literacy approach. *Communication Education*, 59(3): 312–27.

Villagran, M., Goldsmith, J., Wittenberg-Lyles, E., and Baldwin, P. (2010). Creating COMFORT: A communication-based model for breaking bad news. *Communication Education*, 59(3): 220–35.

von Friederichs-Fitzwater, M., and Gilgun, J. (2001). Relational control in physician–patient encounters [Special issue]. *Health Communication*, 13: 75–87.

von Gunten, C.F. (2002). Secondary and tertiary palliative care in U.S. hospitals. *Journal of the American Medical Association*, 286: 875–81.

Wagner, M. (2010, February). Skype helping dementia patients, families stay in touch. Computer World. Retrieved Feb 12, 2010, from: <http://blogs.computerworld.com>.

Wagner, P., Hendrich, J., Moseley, G., and Hudson, V. (2007). Defining medical professionalism: A qualitative study. *Medical Education*, 41: 288–94.

Walker, K. L., Arnold, C. L., Miller-Day, M., and Webb, L. M. (2001). Investigating the physician–patient relationship: examining emerging themes. *Health Communication*, 14(1): 45–68.

Walker, L., Kohler, R., Heys, S., and Eremin, O. (1998). Psychosocial aspects of cancer in the elderly. *European Journal of Surgical Oncology*, 24: 375–8.

Wallack, L. (1989). Mass communication and health promotion: A critical perspective. In R. E. Rice and C. K. Atkin (eds), *Public Communication Campaigns* (2nd edn, pp. 353–67). Newbury Park, CA: Sage.

Wallis, C. (2009, November 2). *A Powerful Identity, a Vanishing Diagnosis*. The New York Times. Retrieved from: <http://www.nytimes.com/2009/11/03/health/03asperger.html>.

Walsh, D., and Gordon, S. (2001). The terminally ill: Dying for palliative medicine? *American Journal of Hospice and Palliative Care*, 18: 203–5.

Walsh-Burke, K. (1992). Family communication and coping with cancer. Impact of the We Can Weekend. *Journal of Psychosocial Oncology*, 10: 63–81.

Wanzer, M., Booth-Butterfield, M. and Gruber, K. (2004). Perceptions of healthcare providers' communication: Relationships between patient-centered communication and satisfaction. *Health Communication*, 16: 363–84.

Wanzer, M., Frymier, A. B., and Sparks, L. (2009). The function of communication within the lives of older adults: An exploration of the relationships among humor, coping efficacy, age, and life satisfaction. *Health Communication*.

Webb, J., et al. (2008). Patient-centered approach for improving prescription drug warning labels. *Patient Education and Counseling*, 72: 443–9.

Weber, B. A., Roberts, B. L., and McDougall, G. J. (2000). Exploring the efficacy of support groups of men with prostate cancer. *Geriatric Nursing*, 41: 250–3.

Weick, K. E. (1969). *The Social Psychology of Organizing*. Reading, MA: Addison-Wesley.

Weiman, J. M. (1977). Explication and test of a model of communicative competence. *Human Communication Research*, 3: 195–213.

Weinberg, N., Schmale, J. D., Uken, J., and Wessel, K. (1995). Computer-mediated support groups. *Social Work with Groups*, 17(4): 43–54.

Weinstein, N. D. (1988). The precaution adoption process. *Health Psychology*, 7: 355–86.

Weinstein, N. D. (1999). What does it mean to understand a risk? Evaluating risk comprehension. *Journal of the National Cancer Institute Monographs*, 25: 15–20.

Weinstein, N. D., and Sandman, P. M. (2002). The precaution adoption process model. In K. Glanz, B. K. Rimer, and F. M. Lewis (eds), *Health Behavior and Health Education: Theory, Research, and Practice* (3rd edn, pp. 121–43). San Francisco, CA: Jossey-Bass.

Weinstein, N. D., Rothman, A., and Sutton, S. (1998). Stage theories of health behavior. *Health Psychology*, 17: 290–9.

Weiss, B. D. (2007). Health literacy and patient safety: Help patients understand. *American Medical Association Manual for Clinicians* (2nd edn). Retrieved from: <http://www.ama–assn.org/ama1/pub/upload/mm/367/healthlitclinicians.pdf>.

Weiss, B. D., et al. (2005). Quick assessment of literacy in primary care: The newest vital sign. *Annals of Family Medicine*, 3(6): 514.

Weitzner, M. A., McMillan, S. C., and Jacobson, P. B. (1999). Family caregiver quality of life: Differences between curative and palliative cancer treatment settings. *Journal of Pain and Symptom Management*, 17: 418–28.

Welbourne, J. L., Blanchard, A. L., and Boughton, M. D. (2009). Supportive communication, sense of virtual community and health outcomes in online infertility groups. *Communities and Technologies*, 1: 31–40.

Wensinga, M., et al. (1999). Systematic review of the literature on patient priorities for general practice care. *Social Science and Medicine*, 47: 1573–88.

Wentz, L. (2009, September 19). Hispanic creative advertising awards 2009 [Web log message]. Retrieved from: <http://adage.com/hispanicawards09/article?article_id=139087>.

Wenzel, L., et al. (2005). Quality of life in long-term cervical cancer survivors. *Gynecologic Oncology*, 97: 310–11.

Whalen, S., and Cheney, G. (1991). Contemporary social theory and its implications for rhetorical and communication theory. *Quarterly Journal of Speech*, 77: 467–79.

Whaley, B. B. (ed.). (2000). *Explaining Illness: Research, Theory, and Strategies*. Mahwah, NJ: Lawrence Erlbaum.

Whelan, T., et al. (2004). Effect of a decision aid on knowledge and treatment decision making for breast cancer surgery. *Journal of the American Medical Association*, 292: 435–41.

The White House (2009). *Health Care*. Retrieved from: <http://www.whitehouse.gov/Issues/health-Care>.

Wiemann, J. M. (1977). Explication and test of a model of communicative competence. *Human Communication Research*, 3: 195–213.

Williams, A., and Nussbaum, J. F. (2001). *Intergenerational Communication across the Lifespan*. Mahwah, NJ: Lawrence Erlbaum.

Williams, C. C. (2008). Insight, stigma, and post-diagnosis identities in schizophrenia. *Psychiatry*, 71: 246–55.

Williams, C. C., and Collins, A. (2002). Factors associated with insight among outpatients with serious mental illness. *Psychiatric Services*, 53: 96–8.

Williams, D. R., and House, J. S. (1991). Stress, social support, control, and coping: A social epidemiologic view. In B. Badura and I. Kickbusch (eds), *Health Promotion Research: Towards a New Social Epidemiology* (pp. 157–72). Copenhagen: World Health Organization.

Williams, D. R., Neighbors, H. W., and Jackson, J. S. (2008). Racism and health: Racial/ethnic bias and health. *American Journal of Public Health*, 98: S29–S37.

Williams, D. R., Spencer, M. S., and Jackson, J. S. (1999). Race, stress, and physical health: The role of group identity. In R. J. Contrada and R. D. Ashmore (eds), *Self, Social Identity, and Physical Health: Interdisciplinary Explorations* (pp. 71–100). New York: Oxford University Press.

Williams, M. V., Davis, T., Parker, R. M., and Weiss, B. D. (2002). The role of health literacy in patient–physician communication. *Family Medicine*, 34: 383–9.

Wills, T. A. (1985). Supportive functions of interpersonal relationships. In S. Cohen and S. L. Syme (eds), *Social Support and Health* (pp. 61–82). New York: Academic Press.

Willyard, J., Miller, K., Shoemaker, M., and Addison, P. (2008). Making sense of sibling responsibility for family caregiving. *Qualitative Health Research*, 18: 1673–86.

Winker, M. A., and Flanagin, A. (1999). Caring for patients at the end of life: Call for papers. *Journal of the American Medical Association*, 282: 1695.

Witte, K. (1992a). Putting the fear back into fear appeals: The extended parallel process model. *Communication Monographs*, 59: 329–49.

Witte, K. (1992b). Preventing AIDS through persuasive communications: A framework for constructing effective, culturally-specific, preventive health messages. *International and Intercultural Communication Annual*, 16: 67–86.

Witte, K. (1994). Generating effective risk messages: How scary should your risk communication be? *Communication Yearbook*, 18: 229–54.

Witte, K. (1998). Fear as motivator, fear as inhibitor: Using the extended parallel process model to explain fear appeal successes and failures. In P. A. Andersen and L. K. Guerrero (eds), *Communication and Emotion: Theory, Research, and Applications* (pp. 424–51). Burlington, MA: Academic Press/Elsevier.

Witte, K., Meyer, G., and Martell, D. (2001). *Effective Health Risk Messages*. Thousand Oaks, CA: Sage.

Witte, K., et al. (1993). Preventing tractor-related injuries and deaths in rural populations: Using a Persuasive Health Message (PHM) framework in formative evaluation research. *International Quarterly of Community Health Education*, 13: 219–51.

Witte, K., Stokols, D., Ituarte, P., and Schneider, M. (1993). Testing the health belief model in a field study to promote bicycle safety helmets. *Communication Research*, 20: 564–86.

Wittenberg-Lyles, E. M. (2005). Information sharing in interdisciplinary team meetings: An evaluation of hospice goals. *Qualitative Health Research*, 15(10): 1377–91.

Wittenberg-Lyles, E. M. (2007). Narratives of hospice volunteers: Perspectives on death and dying. *Qualitative Research Reports*, 7(1): 1–6.

Wittenberg-Lyles, E. M., Goldsmith, J., Sanchez-Reilly, S., Ragan, S., (2008) Communicating a terminal prognosis in a palliative care setting: deficiencies in current communication training protocols. *Social Science & Medicine*, 66: 2356–65.

Wittenberg-Lyles, E. M., Villagran, M. M., & Hajek, C. (2008). Communicating about advance directives: Cultural differences between Latinos and European-Americans. *Journal of Ethnic and Cultural Diversity in Social Work*, 349–364.

Wolf, M. S., Chang, C. H., Davis, T. and Makoul, G. (2005). Development and validation of the Communication and Attitudinal Self-Efficacy Scale for cancer (CASE-cancer). *Patient Education and Counseling*, 57: 333–41.

Wolf, M. S., Gazmararian, J. A., and Baker, D. W. (2007). Health literacy and health risk behaviors among older adults. *American Journal of Preventive Medicine*, 32: 19–24.

Wolf, M. S., Parker, R. M., and Ratzan, S. C. (2008). Literacy and public health. *International Encyclopedia of Public Health* (pp. 98–104). Amsterdam: Elsevier.

Word, C. O., Zanna, M. P., and Cooper, J. (1974). The nonverbal mediation of self-fulfilling prophecies in interracial interaction. *Journal of Experimental Social Psychology*, 10: 109–20.

World Health Organization (2009). *Gender*. Retrieved from: <http://www.who.int/topics/gender/en/>.

Wortman, C., and Dunkel-Schetter, C. (1979). Interpersonal relationships and cancer. *Journal of Social Issues*, 35: 120–55.

Wright, K. B. (1997). Shared ideology in Alcoholic Anonymous: A grounded theory approach. *Journal of Health Communication*, 2: 83–99.

Wright, K. B. (2000). The communication of social support within an on-line community for older adults: A qualitative analysis of the SeniorNet community. *Qualitative Research Reports in Communication*, 1: 33–43.

Wright, K. B. (2002). Social support within an on-line cancer community: An assessment of emotional support, perceptions of advantages and disadvantages, and motives for using the community from a communication perspective. *Journal of Applied Communication Research*, 30: 195–209.

Wright, K. B., and Bell, S. B. (2003). Health-related support groups on the Internet: Linking empirical findings to social support and computer–mediated communication theory. *Journal of Health Psychology*, 8: 37–52.

Wright, K. B., Sparks, L., and O'Hair, H. D. (2008). *Health Communication in the 21st Century*. Oxford: Blackwell.

Wykle, M. L., and Ford, A. B. (1999). *Serving Minority Elders in the 21st Century*. New York: Springer.

Yalom, I. (1995). *The Theory and Practice of Group Psychotherapy.* New York: Basic Books.

Yang, L. H., et al. (2007). Culture and stigma: Adding moral experience to stigma theory. *Social Science and Medicine,* 64: 1524–35.

Yeo, G., and Hikoyeda, N. (2000). Cultural issues in end-of-life decision making among Asians and Pacific Islanders in the United States. In K. L. Braun, J. H. Pietsch, and P. L. Blanchette (eds), *Cultural Issues in End-of-Life Decision Making* (pp. 101–125). Thousand Oaks, CA: Sage.

Young, A. J., and Rodriguez, K. L. (2006). The role of narrative in discussing end-of-life care: Eliciting values and goals from text, context, and subtext. *Health Communication,* 19(1): 49–59.

Zamborsky, L. J. (1996). Support groups for hospice staff. In D. C. Sheehan and W. B. Forman (eds), *Hospice and Palliative Care: Concepts and Practices* (pp. 131–7). Sudbury, MA: Jones and Bartlett Publishers.

Zerzan, J., Stearns, S., and Hanson, L. (2000). Access to palliative care and hospice in nursing homes. *Journal of the American Medical Association,* 284: 2489–94.

Zietlow, P. H., and Sillars, A. L. (1988). Life-stage differences in communication during marital conflicts. *Journal of Social and Personal Relationships,* 5: 223–45.

Zimmerman, S., and Applegate, J. L. (1992). Person-centered comforting in the hospice interdisciplinary team. *Communication Research,* 19: 240–63.

Zoppi, K., and Epstein, R. M. (2002). Is communication a skill? Communication behaviors and being in relation. *Family Medicine,* 34(5): 319–24.

Index